NEUROPATHOLOGY REVIEW

Neuropathology Review

By
Richard A. Prayson, MD
Department of Anatomic Pathology
Cleveland Clinic Foundation, Cleveland, OH

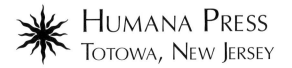 Humana Press
Totowa, New Jersey

For additional copies, pricing for bulk purchases, and/or information about other Humana titles, contact Humana at the above address or at any of the following numbers: Tel.: 973-256-1699; Fax: 973-256-8341; E-mail:humana@humanapr.com; Website: http://humanapress.com

Cover illustrations: Inset gross picture depicts a brain with lissencephaly. The background microscopic picture is of subacute sclerosing panencephalitis. Artwork courtesy of Richard A. Prayson, MD.
Cover design by Patricia F. Cleary.

This publication is printed on acid-free paper. ∞
ANSI Z39.48-1984 (American National Standards Institute) Permanence of Paper for Printed Library Materials.

Printed in the United States of America. 10 9 8 7 6 5 4 3 2 1

Library of Congress Cataloging-in-Publication Data

Prayson, Richard A.
        Neuropathology review / by Richard A. Prayson.
                 p.   ;cm.
        Includes bibliographical references and index.
        ISBN 1-58829-024-7 (alk. paper)
        1. Nervous system—Diseases—Outline, syllabi, etc. . 2. Nervous system—Diseases—Examinations, questions, etc. I. Title.
        [DNLM: 1. Nervous System Diseases—Outlines. WL 18.2 P921n 2001]
        RC347.P724 2001
        616.8'0076—dc21   2001016673

PREFACE

The scope of neuropathology continues to expand, as evidenced by increasing numbers of multivolume and specialty texts that have been published in recent years. For those in the neuroscience disciplines, the ever increasing amount of information one needs to assimilate and master can be challenging and even at times daunting.

Neuropathology Review attempts to summarize, in outline form, the essentials of neuropathology. The objective is twofold: (1) to provide an overview of neuropathology, for those initially encountering the discipline and, (2) to provide a framework for review for those preparing for in-service and board examinations in the disciplines of neurology, neurosurgery, and pathology that require some knowledge of neuropathology.

The text is divided into three main sections. The first part (Chapters 1–11) presents, in outline form, basic information on the spectrum of neurologic-related disease. The second part (Chapters 12 and 13) will present pertinent pictorial examples of a spectrum of neuropathologic conditions in a question format with answers and brief explanation provided. The final section (Chapters 14 and 15) will include a series of written questions provided with answers and explanations in order to review the material presented in the first section of the text.

The author would like to thank Ms. Denise Egleton for her help in preparing this manuscript and to acknowledge Dr. Caroline Abramovich for her review of the text.

Richard A. Prayson, MD

CONTENTS

1 Normal Histology

I. Central Nervous System

  A. Neurons

- 5–100 µm in size
- Variety of shapes: stellate, oval, round, pyramidal, bipolar and unipolar
- Nucleus
  - Vesicular with prominent nucleolus
  - Scalloped—Purkinje cells and pyramidal cells in cortical layer V
- Cytoplasm
  - Mitochondria prominent
  - Nissl substance—granular basophilic material, rough endoplasmic reticulum
  - Neurofilaments (60–100 Å, transport function)
  - May have pigments such as lipofuscin and melanin
- Cell processes
  - Axon—conducts away from cell body, arises from axon hillock which contains no Nissl substance; axoplasm with mitochondria, neurotubules, and neurofilaments
  - Dendrite—conducts toward cell body, contains Nissl substance
- Pigmented (neuromelanin) neurons—coarse, dark brown granules
  - Substantia nigra (midbrain)
  - Locus ceruleus (pons)
  - Dorsal motor nucleus of the vagus nerve (medulla)
- Synaptophysin immunostain positive—membrane protein of synaptic vesicles
- Lipofuscin (aging pigment, lipochrome)
  - Increases with age
  - Intracytoplasmic
  - Light yellow-brown color on routine hematoxylin and eosin staining
- Hyaline (colloid inclusion)
  - Cytoplasmic
  - Endoplasmic reticulum dilated cisternae
- Marinesco bodies
  - Eosinophilic intranuclear inclusions
  - May be multiple within one nucleus
  - Prominently seen in pigmented neurons
  - Increases with age
- A variety of other inclusions within neurons may be seen in association with certain disease processes (e.g., Lewy bodies, tangles, Hirano bodies, Pick bodies, granulovacuolar degeneration, viral inclusions, etc.)
- Ischemic changes—"red and dead"—shrunken cell body with dark nucleus, indistinguishable nucleolus, and eosinophilic cytoplasm.
- Central chromatolysis—related to axonal or retrograde degeneration, cytoplasmic swelling with loss of Nissl substance, and peripheralization/flattening of the nucleus, may be reversible to a point
- Ferruginization of neurons (fossilized neurons)—encrusted with calcium and/or iron, may be seen in old infarcts.

- Neuronophagia—phagocytosis of cell body
- Axonal spheroids—focal dilatation of axon with neurofilaments and organelles, reaction to axon injury, Purkinje cell axonal spheroids called torpedoes

B. Astrocytes
- Largest of glial cells
- Vesicular nucleus without nucleolus
- Cytoplasm highlighted with GFAP (glial fibrillary acidic protein) antibody
- Processes often invest vessels
- A variety of shapes
  - Star-shaped fibrillary (white matter) and protoplasmic (gray matter) cells
  - Pilocytic astrocytes of periventricular region and cerebellum
  - Bergmann astrocytes of cerebellum
- Corpora amylacea
  - Laminated, basophilic polyglucosan bodies
  - Associated with astrocytic foot processes
  - Increase with age
  - Frequently seen in subpial regions
- Reactive astrocytes (gemistocytes)
  - Cell hypertrophy—increased cell cytoplasm
  - Gliosis may be associated with increased cell number
- Rosenthal fiber
  - Cytoplasmic inclusion
  - Brightly eosinophilic, elongated structures
  - Observed in a number of entities including gliosis, Alexander's disease, pilocytic astrocytoma
- Creutzfeldt astrocyte
  - Reactive astrocytes with multiple small nuclei
  - Seen in demyelinative processes
- Alzheimer type I astrocyte
  - Large cells often with multiple nuclei or irregularly lobulated nuclei
  - Seen in progressive multifocal leukoencephalopathy

- Alzheimer type II astrocyte
  - Nuclear swelling and chromatin clearing
  - Prominent nucleolation
  - Cell cytoplasm not readily apparent
  - Prominently seen in globus pallidus in hepatic diseases that produce elevated ammonia levels
- Viral inclusions in astrocytes
  - Cowdry A—intranuclear, eosinophilic, or basophilic viral inclusion; displaces the nucleolus (e.g., subacute sclerosing panencephalitis (SSPE), progressive multifocal leukoencepholopathy (PML), herpes, cytomegalovirus (CMV)
  - Cowdry B—intranuclear, eosinophilic viral inclusion; often multiple and smaller than Cowdry A inclusions, generally do not displace the nucleolus (e.g., polio)

C. Oligodendrocytes
- Most numerous cells in the central nervous system (CNS)
- Small cells with no cytoplasmic staining with hematoxylin and eosin
- Thinner and fewer cell processes than astrocytes
- Tend to arrange themselves around neurons (neuronal satellitosis)
- "Fried egg" appearance is a delayed postformalin-fixation artifact (will not be seen at frozen section)
- Cells often arranged in small rows in the white matter between myelinated fibers
- Involved in the formation and maintenance of myelin
- Only weak immunostaining with GFAP, positive staining with S-100 protein antibody
- May contain intranuclear inclusions in PML and SSPE.

D. Ependyma
- Epithelioid cells that line ventricular walls and central canal of the spinal cord
- Columnar/cuboidal cells with cilia
- Cilia attached to cell body by blepharoplast
- Ependyma-lined central canal is patent in childhood but generally becomes obliterated at puberty

- Ependymal loss with injury accompanied by a proliferation of subependymal glia (granular ependymitis)

E. Microglia
- Small, dark, elongated nuclei with scant cytoplasm
- HAM56 positive
- May proliferate in a diffuse pattern (microgliosis) or nodular pattern (microglial nodule)—commonly seen with viral encephalitis
- With destruction of parenchymal tissue, will see a macrophage response (gitter cells)
- Macrophages seen in a variety of pathologies (e.g., infarct, demyelinating disease, radiation, abscess)

F. Choroid plexus
- Produces cerebrospinal fluid (CSF), usually intraventricular in location
- May see choroid plexus in subarachnoid space in cerebellopontine angle region
- Fibrovascular cores lined by epithelial cells, cobblestoned contour
- May see small nests of arachnoidal (meningothelial) cells intermixed
- May be focally calcified

G. Arachnoid cap cells
- Seen principally in the arachnoid membrane
- Associated with psammoma body formation (laminated calcifications)
- Dorsal leptomeninges of cord may contain white firm plaques (arachnoiditis ossificans)—laminated dense hyalinized fibrous tissue
- May see melanocytes in the meninges, more prominent in darker skinned individuals
- Dura overlying the leptomeninges comprised primarily of dense fibrous connective tissue

H. Architecture
- Cortex
  - Six layers, parallel to surface
  - Neurons within the layers have their processes oriented perpendicular to the surface
  - Layers
    I. Molecular—few small neurons, glia, outermost layer
    II. External granular—small neurons with short axons
    III. Outer pyramidal—medium and large neurons
    IV. Internal granular—small stellate neurons
    V. Inner pyramidal—medium size neurons, Betz cells
    VI. Polymorphic layer—innermost layer
- Cerebellum
  - Three layers
    ▶ Molecular layer—outermost layer
    ▶ Purkinje cell layer—single layer of neurons
    ▶ Granular cell layer—hypercellular, small cells
  - Outer granular cell layer in infant overlies molecular layer, disappears by age 1 yr
- White matter
  - Fibers run at right angles to cortical surface
  - Includes centrum semiovale
  - Two bundles in gray matter parallel to surface
    ▶ Inner line of Baillarger between layers 3 and 4
    ▶ Stria of Gennari between layers 5 and 6 in occipital lobe
- Basal ganglia
  - Includes caudate, putamen, globus pallidus, and amygdala
  - Gray matter tissue
  - Caudate and putamen contain thin fascicles of myelinated fibers (pencil bundles of Wilson)
- Hippocampus
  - Consists of dentate gyrus, Ammon's horn, and subiculum
  - Ammon's horn (CA = cornu Ammon's) divided into four regions
    ▶ CA4 endplate region within the hilus of the dentate gyrus
    ▶ CA3 connects endplate to resistance sector (CA2)

▶ CA1 Sommer sector (most sensitive area of brain to anoxic damage)

- Spinal cord
  - Enlargement of anterior (ventral) horns in cervical and lumbosacral region
  - Central canal in middle
  - Terminates with filum terminale
- Pineal gland
  - Vaguely nodular architectural arrangement of cells with glial background
  - Corpora arenacea—calcifications, present after puberty
  - Pineal cysts—gliotic cysts often with Rosenthal fibers
- Pituitary gland
  - Adenohypophysis—nests of epithelioid cells separated by delicate fibrovascular septae, cell types in a given nest are mixed type, geographic predominance of certain cell types
  - Pars intermedia—at interface between adenohypophysis and neurohypophysis, glandular formations may be seen
  - Neurohypophysis—spindled cells loosely arranged

II. Skeletal Muscle

A. Muscle fibers arranged in bundles (fascicles) surrounded by perimysium connective tissue; endomysium is connective tissue between muscle fibers

B. Nuclei multiple, peripherally arranged
  - Central nuclei abnormal if seen in >3–5% of myofibers;
  - Increased central nuclei in myotonic dystrophy, myotubular myopathy, Charcot-Marie-Tooth disease

C. At muscle–tendon junction, fibers get smaller and often contain internalized nuclei.

D. In cross section, fibers are generally the same size
  - Atrophy
    - Scattered versus grouped (neurogenic), tend to have angulated contours
    - Rounded fiber atrophy—more likely myopathic

  - Perifascicular atrophy—ischemia related, characteristic of dermatomyositis
  - Fascicular atrophy—spinal muscular atrophy, hereditary motor and sensory neuropathies, vasculitis
  - Type I atrophy—myotonic dystrophy, congenital myopathies, spinocerebellar degeneration
  - Type II atrophy—disuse, steroids (type IIB), collagen vascular disease, myasthenia gravis, cachexia, paraneoplastic neuromyopathy
- Hypertrophy
  - Normal in athletes (type II fibers)
  - Often associated with central nuclei and split fibers.

E. Muscle fiber types (type I, type IIA, type IIB) generally distributed in a mosaic/checkerboard pattern
  - Type I fibers—high oxidative, low glycolytic activity
  - Type II fibers—low oxidative, high glycolytic activity
  - Different muscles contain different proportions of the three fiber types
  - Loss of the mosaic distribution of fiber types—fiber type grouping, indicative of chronic denervation and reinnervation

F. Muscle cells of variable length—run from origin to insertion

G. Muscle cells made up of myofilaments
  - Two main types: thick myosin filaments and thin actin filaments
  - Sarcomere segment is the functional contractile unit of muscle formed by the orderly arrangement of myofilaments
  - Sarcomeric banding patterns
    - Dark central A (anisotropic) band consisting of mostly thick myosin filaments
    - A band crossed at midpoint by a dark narrow transverse M line consisting of crossbridges which link adjacent, myosin filaments together
    - M band surrounded by paler H band which varies in width as the sarcomeric length changes

- Pale I (isotropic) band situated on either side of the A band consisting mostly of thin, actin filaments in combination with troponin and tropomyosin proteins

- Z band divides I band at midpoint and marks the longitudinal boundary of each sarcomere

- During contraction of the fiber, I filaments slide toward the center of the A band with shortening of the I and H bands

- Desmin intermediate filaments link Z discs together and join them to the plasmalemma

H. Sarcoplasm

- Represents the cytoplasm of the myofiber

- Consists of a variety of structures/organelles

  - Mitochondria—type I > type II

  - T system (transverse tubular system)—network of tubules which is continuous with the muscle cell plasma membrane, allows for the rapid passage of depolarization into the interior of the myofiber

  - Sarcoplasmic reticulum—a series of flattened sacs between and around myofbrils

  - Lipid—droplets lie between myofibrils and adjacent to mitochondria, type I > type II

  - Glycogen—more prominent in region of I band than A band, type II > type I

  - Ribosomes, Golgi membranes, intermediate filaments, microtubules, and lipofuscin also seen.

I. Muscle spindle

- Collections of small intrafusal fibers (3–14) enclosed in a connective tissue capsule

- Center of spindle is swollen, ends are tapered

- Located between muscle fascicles in perimysial connective tissue

- Consists of two types of intrafusal fibers: nuclear bag fibers and nuclear chain fibers

- More numerous in muscles involved in delicate movements

- Associated with sensory nerve endings

J. Motor unit—consists of anterior horn cell, nerve fiber arising from it and the muscle fibers supplied by it.

K. Neuromuscular junction—interface between the nerve and muscle, acetylcholine is released by the nerve to activate the muscle; the electrical impulse reaches the sarcoplasmic reticulum via the T system.

III. Peripheral Nerve

A. Connective tissue layers

- Epineurium—binds fascicles together, continuous with dura mater at junction of spinal nerves and spinal nerve roots

- Perineurium—concentric layers of flattened cells which are epithelial membrane antigen (EMA) positive, separated by collagen that surrounds individual fascicles, forms part of the blood–nerve barrier, continuous with the pia arachnoid

- Endoneurium—collagen compartment that surrounds individual axons, Schwann cells, and fibroblasts

B. Mast cells also present in endoneurium, increase in number with axonal degeneration and neurofibroma

C. Renaut bodies–cylindrical hyaline bodies attached to inner aspect of the perineurium; composed of collagen fibers, fibroblasts and epineurial cells; function not known, increase in number in compressive neuropathies.

D. Blood supply comes from vasa nervorum

E. Nerve fibers

- Either myelinated or unmyelinated

- Class A fibers

  - Myelinated

  - 1–20 μm in diameter; conduction velocity 12–100 m/s

- Class B fibers

  - Myelinated preganglionic autonomic fibers

  - Up to 3 μm in diameter; conduction velocity 3–15 m/s

- Class C fibers

  - Unmyelinated

  - Small fibers (0.2–1.5 μm diameter); conduction velocity 0.3–1.6 m/s

F. Myelin

- Can be highlighted with certain stains (Luxol fast blue, Loyez, osmium, periodic acid schiff (PAS), Masson trichrome)

- Formed by fusion of Schwann cell membranes
- 75% lipid and 25% protein
- Major lipids comprising myelin: cholesterol, sphingomyelin, galactolipid
- One Schwann cell per myelinated axon (in CNS, one oligodendrocyte supplies myelin to multiple axons)
- Schwann cells S-100 positive by immunohistochemistry
- Pi granules of Reich—lamellated structures, cytoplasm accumulates along with lipofuscin with increasing age
- Corpuscles of Erzholz—spherical bodies in Schwann cell cytoplasm.

G. Schmidt-Lanterman clefts
- Cleft splits the cytoplasmic membranes and serves as a route of passage for substances from the outer cytoplasmic layer through the myelin sheath to the inner cytoplasm
- The number of clefts correlate with the diameter of the axon

H. Node of Ranvier
- Gaps in the myelin sheath

- Distance between nodes is proportional to myelin thickness
- Conduction of impulses along myelinated fibers proceeds in a discontinuous manner from node to node (saltatory conduction)

I. Myelinated axons
- Axon delimited by axolemma membrane
- Axolemma separated from adjacent Schwann cell by periaxonal space of Klebs
- Axonal cytoplasm contains mitochondria, smooth endoplasmic reticulum, glycogen, ribosomes, peroxisomes, neurotransmitter vesicles, and filaments/tubules
- Filaments include actin, neurofilaments, and microtubules

J. Unmyelinated axons
- Best evaluated and studied by electron microscopy
- More numerous than myelinated axons: 3–4 : 1 unmyelinated : myelinated axons
- Frequently associated with Schwann cells; may be more than one axon per Schwann cell

2 Vascular Lesions

I. Anoxia

  A. Anoxia observed in a wide variety of clinical conditions and forms

- Anoxic anoxia—insufficient oxygen reaches blood (e.g., drowning)

- Anemic anoxia—insufficient oxygen content in blood (e.g., carbon monoxide poisoning)

- Histotoxic anoxia—poisons interfere with oxygen utilization (e.g., cyanide, sulfide)

- Stagnant anoxia—most common, decreased cerebral perfusion (e.g., cardiac arrest); factors that determine amount of brain damage after cardiac arrest include duration of ischemia, degree of ischemia, temperature during the event and blood glucose levels

  B. Precise mechanisms not completely elucidated; however, a number of consequences occur which have a negative effect on the CNS

- Edema

- Lactic acid accumulation, decreased pH

- Increase in free fatty acids

- Increase in extracellular potassium and ammonia

- Abnormalities in calcium flux

- Reperfusion problems

  C. Morphology of ischemia highly variable and unpredictable.

- Numerous regional and cellular vulnerabilities exist; the entire brain not uniformly involved (selective vulnerability)

- Neurons most sensitive to anoxia

    ○ Hippocampal, Sommer sector (CA1) most sensitive

    ○ Cerebral cortex, layers III, V, and VI (which contain larger-size neurons)

    ○ Cerebellar Purkinje cells (if patient survives for a period of time, may see Bergmann gliosis)

    ○ Caudate and putamen

- Accentuated in the boundary zones between vascular distributions

  D. Gross pathology

- Swollen, soft

- Gray matter is dusky

- Areas of cavitation in a laminar pattern may be observed

    ○ Pseudolaminar is used to describe involvement of more than one cortical layer

    ○ Laminar describes involvement of a single cortical layer

  E. Microscopic pathology

- Dendrite and astrocyte swelling (i.e., sponginess of the neuropil)

- Ischemic (homogenized) neurons (i.e., "red and dead")

- Endothelial hyperplasia

- Microglial reaction

- Dissolution of neurons after several days

II. Infarction

A. General

- Cerebral blood flow 20% of cardiac output, 15% of oxygen consumption of body.

- Main anterior flow (70%) through internal carotid arteries; posterior flow via vertebral arteries—these systems anastomose via the anterior and posterior communicating arteries to form the circle of Willis

- Disruption in flow can result in infarct (stroke)

- Stroke is a clinical term referring to "abrupt onset of focal or global neurological symptoms caused by ischemia or hemorrhage"—symptoms >24 h; if symptoms resolve in less than 24 h = transient ischemic attack (TIA)

- Risk of stroke increased with increasing age, male > female, smoking, hypertension, atrial fibrillation, carotid artery stenosis, hyperlipidemia, diabetes, heart surgery, antiphospholipid antibodies, high-estrogen oral contraceptives

- Venous thrombosis associated with pregnancy and oral contraceptive use

   o Most common sites of venous thrombosis in superior sagittal sinus, lateral sinuses, and straight sinus

   o Septic thrombosis most common in cavernous sinus, often due to contiguous spread from soft tissue/sinus infection

B. Determining the age of an infarct either grossly or microscopically can only be done within a wide range. The times given are guidelines rather than absolutes.

C. Gross pathology

- Unequivocal alterations require up to 24 h; early changes include edema, congestion, softening

- 48 h: "cracking"—separation of the necrotic tissue from intact tissue

- 72 h: infarcted area usually clearly delineated; cortex friable and soft

- A 1-cm cavity takes 2–3 months to form

- Once cavitation begins, it is difficult to determine the age of the infarct.

D. Microscopic pathology

- Earliest changes: (1) astrocytic swelling, (2) interstitial edema, (3) pyknosis, (4) hypereosinophilia of neurons, (5) microvacuolization of neurons (swollen mitochondria)

- 24 h: macrophage infiltration begins, axonal swelling, may see neutrophilic infiltration (ceases by d 5)

- 3–4 d: prominent macrophage infiltration

- 7–10 d: astrocytic proliferation and hypertrophy evident

- 30 d: intense gliosis

- May have a hemorrhagic component (18–48%); most hemorrhagic infarcts are embolic artery events; hemorrhage in infarcts due to reperfusion of necrotic vessels or occlusion of venous drainage

- May encounter degeneration of tracts distal to infarct

E. Lacunar infarct

- The infarcts range in size from 3–4 mm up to 1.5 cm

- Most common sites: putamen, caudate, thalamus, pons, internal capsule, and convolutional white matter

- Causes: (1) lipohyalinosis, (2) occlusion of small penetrating vessels, (3) dissection, (4) emboli

- Small perivascular cavities common in basal ganglia and deep white matter; état lacunairé (gray matter) and état criblé (deep white matter)

F. Respirator brain

- Also known as (AKA) diffuse anoxic encephalopathy

- Permanent global ischemia due to nonperfusion of entire brain

- Brain perfusion depends on mean arterial blood pressure exceeding the intracranial pressure (cerebral perfusion pressure = mean arterial blood pressure − intracranial pressure)

- The most extreme form of stagnant anoxia

- Grossly—dusky brown discoloration of cortex, blurring of gray–white junction, general friability of tissue (brain often does not fix well in formalin)

- Microscopically—ischemic neurons everywhere ± infarcts

G. Carbon monoxide (CO) poisoning
- A form of anemic anoxia due to displacement of oxygen from its binding site on hemoglobin
- CO binds irreversibly to hemoglobin, reducing its oxygen-carrying capacity
- CO directly binds to iron-rich areas of brain (globus pallidus and pars reticulata of substantia nigra)
- Pathologically marked by necrosis of globus pallidus and substantia nigra.
- May see demyelination and cerebral white matter destruction (Grenker's myelinopathy)

H. Air embolism
- May be related to decompression sickness "the bends"—nitrogen gas in blood, can cause spinal cord microinfarcts
- May also occur related to cardiac bypass surgery

I. Hypoglycemic brain damage
- Causes selective neuronal necrosis-like ischemia
- Different mechanism of injury than ischemia
  - Decreased lactate and pyruvate
  - Tissue alkalosis
- Neuronal necrosis in cerebral cortex superficial layers, hippocampus (CA1 and dentate) and caudate; no Purkinje cell necrosis

III. Aneurysms
A. Saccular aneurysms
- AKA: "berry," congenital or medical defect
- Incidence in general population, 2–5%; female : male 3 : 2.
- Usually present at arterial bifurcation; most asymptomatic
  - 85% in anterior circle of Willis
  - 25% multiple
  - 20% bilateral
- Most common sites
  - Middle cerebral artery trifurcation
  - Anterior communicating artery junction
  - Internal carotid artery—posterior communicating artery junction
- Risk of rupture, greatest in aneurysms > 1 cm in size
- "Giant aneurysm" defined as > 2.5 cm, usually causes compressive or embolic symptoms
- Etiology
  - Many theories
  - Congenital defects of part or all of the media at the arterial bifurcation, does not explain why most arise in adulthood
  - Remnants of embryonic vessels
  - Focal destruction of the internal elastic membrane due to hemodynamic alterations, about 3–9% of patients with arteriovenous malformation (AVM) have aneurysms
  - Abnormalities in specific collagen subsets
  - Associated conditions:
    - Polycystic kidney disease, Potter type 3
    - Ehlers–Danlos syndrome (types IV and VI)
    - Coarctation of the aorta
    - Marfan's syndrome
    - Pseudoxanthoma elasticum
- Pathology
  - Media usually defective
  - Intimal hyperplasia and sometimes a gap in the internal elastic membrane seen
  - Aneurysm wall usually contains fibrous tissue
  - Atherosclerotic changes occasionally seen
  - Phagocytosis and hemosiderin deposition may be present

B. Infectious (septic) aneurysms
- Most related to bacterial endocarditis
  - Arterial wall weakened by pyogenic bacteria which usually reach the wall by an infected embolus
  - May be multiple
  - Located on distal branches of the middle cerebral artery

- Organisms usually of low virulence, particularly *Streptococcus viridans* and *Staphylococcus aureus*
- Mycotic aneurysms typically refer to fungal aneurysms; Aspergillus the most common organism responsible

C. Fusiform aneurysms

- Related to dolichoectasia (elongation, widening, and tortuosity of a cerebral artery)
- Supraclinoid segment of internal carotid artery and basilar artery most common sites
- Fusiform aneurysm refers to dilated segment of artery
- Seen commonly with advanced atherosclerosis

IV. Vascular Malformations

A. General information

- True malformations result from the embryonic vascular network
- Some increase in size by incorporating adjacent vessels—"recruitment"
- Clinical symptoms include seizures, "steal" phenomenon, hemorrhage
- In children, excessive shunting may lead to cardiac decompensation (especially vein of Galen malformations).
- True incidence of hemorrhage unknown, estimates = 5–10% overall
- A subset of malformations is of mixed type.

B. Arteriovenous malformation (AVM)

- Admixture of arteries, veins, and intermediate size vessels
- Vessels are separated by gliotic neural parenchyma
- Foci of mineralization and hemosiderin deposition common
- Typically superficial, wedge-shaped with the apex directed toward the ventricle
- Commonly found in surgical series; the most common vascular malformation associated with hemorrhage; peak presentation 2nd–4th decades

C. Venous malformation (angioma)

- Veins of varying sizes
- Vessels separated by mostly "normal" parenchyma
- Less compact than AVM or cavernous malformation
- May have a large central draining vein
- Varix is a single dilated/large vein

D. Cavernous malformation (angioma)

- Large, sinusoidal-type vessels in apposition to each other
- Little or no intervening parenchyma
- Compact malformations
- Mineralization and ossification common; occasionally massive
- May bleed

E. Capillary telangiectasia

- Capillary sized vessels
- Separated by normal neural parenchyma
- Common in the striate pons
- Often an "incidental" finding at autopsy

V. Hemorrhage

A. Common causes

- Spontaneous intracerebral hemorrhage, often ganglionic (caudate, putamen) related to hypertension—most common cause of nontraumatic hemorrhage
- Ruptured saccular aneurysm
- Vascular malformation, particularly AVM and cavernous angioma
- Coagulopathy associated, may have both platelet and prothrombin time abnormalities
- Congophilic (amyloid) angiopathy
  - Lobar hemorrhage
  - Elderly
  - Amyloid deposition in vessel walls both in meninges and cortex
  - Most commonly β-amyloid type (chromosome 21)
  - Associated with Down's syndrome and Alzheimer's disease
  - Highlighted on Congo red (apple green birefringence with polarized light), thioflavin S or T, and crystal violet stains
- Neoplasms
- Blood dyscrasias (i.e., sickle cell anemia)
- Vasculitis

B. Pathology
- Soft, gelatinous clot
- Small vessels with thrombosis may project into the hemorrhage
- Petechial hemorrhage may be seen around the large hemorrhage
- Ischemic necrosis seen in associated brain tissue
- Clot edge often has hemosiderin-laden macrophages
- Astrocytic proliferation often prominent at the edge
- Amyloid may be seen in adjacent vessels if congophilic angiopathy is the cause
- Venous hemorrhage—usually the infarcts are larger and not confined to any arterial distribution, often over the convexity

VI. Vasculitis

A. Common causes
- Polyarteritis nodosa (PAN) and its variants
  - Systemic disease
  - Male : female 2 : 1
  - Any age, peak 40–50 yr
  - Necrotizing vasculitis with fibrinoid necrosis of medium-sized vessels
  - May represent immune-complex-mediated vasculitis (subset of patients are hepatitis B or C positive)
- Hypersensitivity angiitis
- Wegener's granulomatosis
  - Systemic disease often with respiratory tract component
  - Most patients 40–60 yr
  - ANCA (anti-neutrophil cytoplasmic antibodies)—directed against proteinase 3
- Lymphomatoid granulomatosis
- Giant cell arteritis
  - The most common of the granulomatous vasculitides
  - Older patients >50 yr
  - Primary target is extracranial arteries of head, but may involve cerebral vessels
  - Headache, blindness, increased erythrocyte sedimentation rate (ESR)
  - Associated with polymyalgia rheumatica
  - May be a focal process (skip lesions)
  - Lymphoplasmacytic inflammation ± granulomas, fibrous scarring with healing
- Takayasu's arteritis
  - Aortic arch and branches and descending aorta
  - Younger patients (15–40 yr), Oriental females at higher risk
  - Lymphoplasmacytic inflammation of the media with fibrosis, granulomas/giant cells
- Thromboangiitis obliterans
- Vasculitis associated with connective tissue disease, (i.e., systemic lupus erythematosus [SLE], Sjögren's syndrome, Behcet's syndrome
- Churg-Strauss—necrotizing vasculitis with eosinophilia
- Primary angiitis of central nervous system
  - Headaches, multifocal deficits, diffuse encephalopathy
  - Adults (ages 30–50 yr)
  - ESR normal or mildly elevated
  - Biopsy of nondominant temporal tip, including leptomeninges (highest yield), cortex, and white matter recommended
  - Arteries involved more than veins
  - May be granulomatous or nongranulomatous
  - May be complicated by infarct or hemorrhage
- Other causes
  - A variety of other conditions can result in a "vasculitic" pattern of injury pathologically
  - Drugs (e.g., cocaine, amphetamines)
  - Infection (e.g., Treponema, Borrelia, Herpes, HIV, Aspergillus, Mucor)
  - Lymphoproliferative disorders
  - Other (demyelinating disease, atherosclerosis, amyloid, etc.)

B. Pathology
- Segmental inflammation and necrosis of

vascular walls are the common features of the above-listed vasculitides.

- Vasculitis associated with SLE and lymphomatoid granulomatosis are the only two which typically involve brain parenchyma.

- PAN, Wegener's granulomatosis, and giant cell arteritis involve vessels in the subarachnoid space, peripheral nervous system, or the extracranial vessels.

- Neurologic dysfunction in all entities is related to ischemia.

VII. Miscellaneous

A. Binswanger's disease

- Rare condition generally presenting between ages 50–60 yr; evolves over 3–5 yr

- Also called subcortical arteriosclerotic encephalopathy

- Moderate intermittent hypertension and progressive, often profound dementia are features.

- Widespread vascular alterations and white matter changes are seen and readily demonstrated with neuroimaging.

- Ventricular dilatation, often secondary to hydrocephalus *ex vacuo*

- Focal and diffuse myelin loss with associated reactive astrocytosis in the deep hemispheric white matter

- Subcortical arcuate fibers are spared.

- Changes most severe in the temporal and occipital lobes.

- Demyelination is thought to be secondary to reduced perfusion due to arteriosclerosis of small penetrating vessels.

B. CADASIL (Cerebral autosomal dominant arteriopathy with subcortical infarcts and leukoencephalopathy)

- Mutation of notch 3 gene on chromosome 19q12

- Strokes and vascular dementia

- Systemic disorder

- Thickened vessel walls (media and adventitia) with basophilic, PAS-positive granules within smooth muscle cells

- Variable degrees of perivascular atrophy

C. Atherosclerosis/hypertensive angiopathy

- Risk factors: dyslipidemia, hypertension, smoking, diabetes

- Initial atherosclerotic lesion is fatty streak marked by foam cells filled with low-density lipoprotein (LDL) cholesterol.

- Fatty streaks may develop into fibrous plaques (especially develop at outer aspects of arterial bifurcation where laminar flow is disturbed)—connective tissue, smooth muscle cells, foam cells, lymphocytes, necrotic cell debris, and extracellular lipids/cholesterol

- Turbulence caused by plaque may cause further disease progression.

- Complicated plaque results from disruption of endothelium resulting in thrombus formation (risk for occlusion and emboli).

- Hypertensive angiopathy shifts the autoregulation (maintains cerebral blood flow at a constant level between mean arterial pressures of 50–150 mm Hg) curve to the right, raising the lower limit of regulation at which adequate cerebral flow can be maintained.

- Malignant hypertension–acute hypertension

  ○ Diffuse cerebral dysfunction, headache, nausea, vomiting, altered consciousness

  ○ May be the result of pheochromocytoma (release of catecholamine), disseminated vasculitis, eclampsia, rebound drug effect

  ○ Brain edema, focal ischemia, and intracerebral hemorrhage

- Chronic hypertension

  ○ Further worsens atherosclerotic changes in large arteries

  ○ Causes small vessel disease with disruption of blood-brain barrier resulting in basal lamina thickening and reduplication, smooth-muscle degeneration, fibrinoid change (necrosis), and increased collagen deposition (lipohyalinosis—collagenous fibrosis)

  ○ May form Charcot-Bouchard microaneurysms (miliary aneurysms)—dilatations/outpouchings of vessel wall caused by fibrinoid change

D. Moyamoya syndrome

- Defined angiographically by spontaneous

occlusion of the circle of Willis and the presence of abnormal collateralization

- Two peaks of incidence—1st and 4th decades

- Most patients young, <20 yr, females > males

- Hemiparesis and hemorrhage

- Intimal fibroplasia usually without atherosclerotic changes, no inflammation

3 Tumors

I. Astrocytic Neoplasms

  A. Classification schemas (grading) for astrocytomas

- WHO classification
    - Grade I: pilocytic astrocytoma, subependymal giant cell astrocytoma
    - Grade II: well-differentiated diffuse astrocytoma, pleomorphic xanthoastrocytoma
    - Grade III: anaplastic astrocytoma
    - Grade IV: glioblastoma multiforme
- Ringertz classification
    - Low-grade astrocytoma
    - Anaplastic astrocytoma
    - Glioblastoma multiforme
- Daumas-Duport classification (St. Anne-Mayo)

Grade	Criteria
1	0/4
2	1/4
3	2/4
4	3–4/4

(Criteria: mitoses, necrosis, nuclear atypia, endothelial proliferation)

  B. Low-grade astrocytoma

- 20% of all gliomas, 10–15% of all astrocytic tumors
- Incidence: 1.4 new cases/1 million population/yr
- 4th-decade peak
- >90% derived from fibrillary astrocytes
- Arise in white matter
- Frontal lobe>parietal>temporal>occipital
- Noncontrast enhancing, ill-defined region of low density on CT scan
- Seizures, sensorimotor deficits, increased intracranial pressure, altered mentation
- Grossly a solid tumor, infiltrative growth pattern, obliterate gray–white junction, subtle color change (yellow/tan or gray)
- Microscopic
    - Uneven cellularity
    - Rare mitoses
    - Irregular nuclear contours, hyperchromatic nuclei
    - Mild pleomorphism
- May see microcystic change (do not see typically with gliosis)
- Calcification (15%)
- Should not see vascular or endothelial proliferation or necrosis
- GFAP (glial fibrillary acidic protein) positive
    - Intermediate cytoplasmic filaments
    - Also stains ependymomas and choroid plexus tumors
    - Decreased staining in higher-grade tumors
- Electron microscopy
    - Astrocytoma cells marked by cytoplasmic intermediate filaments (7–11 nm)

- ○ Generally not useful for diagnosis
- DNA/cell proliferation
  - ○ Most diploid
  - ○ Ki-67 (MIB-1) proliferation indices roughly correlate with tumor grade
  - ○ Tumor heterogeneity in proliferation—different rates of cell proliferation and varying histologic appearance in different regions of the tumor
- Molecular genetics
  - ○ TP53 mutations in >60% of diffuse astrocytomas (chromosome 17)—appear to progress more frequently
  - ○ Increased platelet-derived growth factor receptor (PDGFR) alpha mRNA expression
  - ○ Other abnormalities which are variably present include gain 7q, amplification 8q, LOH on 10p, and LOH on 22q.
- May remain well differentiated or progress to a higher-grade tumor over time
- Average postoperative survival 6–8 yr
- Young age and gross total resection do better

C. Gemistocytic astrocytoma
- Cells with plump, eosinophilic cell bodies and short processes
- Nuclei usually eccentric with small nucleoli
- Perivascular lymphocytes common
- Lots of gemistocytes associated with more aggressive behavior (20% or more gemistocytic component)
- Gemistocytes usually with lower rate of cell proliferation than background tumor cells

D. Gliosis versus glioma
- Brain tissue adjacent to other lesions may have gliosis
- Limited biopsy makes it difficult to distinguish reactive gliosis from glioma
- Biopsy for recurrent tumor will show reactive gliosis
- History of head trauma—may see gliosis
- Reactive gliosis

- ○ Hypertrophic cells (reactive astrocytes) prominent
- ○ Hypercellularity with even distribution
- ○ Lack nuclear hyperchromasia and angularity
- ○ Absent calcification
- ○ Rosenthal fibers—intensely eosinophilic, elongate, or corkscrew-shaped structures
- ○ Collagen and hemosiderin deposition
- ○ Lack microcystic change
- ○ No satellitosis

 E. Anaplastic astrocytoma
- 4th and 5th decades
- Can arise from low-grade astrocytoma
- Clinical presentation similar to low-grade astrocytoma
- Same gross pathologic features as low-grade astrocytoma
- Microscopic pathology
  - ○ Hypercellularity with more prominent nuclear pleomorphism versus low-grade astrocytoma
  - ○ Mitotic figures more readily identifiable
  - ○ Vascular or endothelial proliferation may be present (not required)—if prominently seen in the tumor, may warrant WHO grade IV designation
  - ○ No necrosis
  - ○ Secondary structures of Sherer (helpful, not always present—satellitosis of tumor cells around pre-existing element such as neurons or vessels)
- Cell proliferation rate greater than low-grade astrocytoma
- P16 deletion (30%), RB alterations (25%), P19 deletion (15%), CDK4 amplification (10%)
- Some with LOH 10q, 19q, and 22q
- Postoperative survival slightly > 2 yr
- Treatment same as glioblastoma multiforme (radiation)

F. Glioblastoma multiforme (GBM)
  - ○ Several possible origins

○ Astrocytic dedifferentiation (associated with a loss of chromosome 10)

○ Nonastrocytic glioma differentiation— some use the term to denote high-grade ependymomas, oligodendrogliomas and mixed gliomas

○ *De novo*—two genetic groups
  ▶ Loss of heterozygosity on chromosome 17p, mutations of *p53* gene, no amplification of epidermal growth factor receptor (EGFR) gene
  ▶ Loss of heterozygosity on chromosome 10 and amplification of EGFR gene; no loss of chromosome 17p

• Tumor suppressor gene loci for astrocytoma on chromosomes 10, 17p, 9p, 19q, and 22

• Most common glioma, 50–60% of all astrocytic neoplasms, 12–15% of all intracranial neoplasms

• 5th and 6th decades

• Rare < age 30 yr

• Male : female 3 : 2

• Increased risks with hydrocarbon exposure and radiation

• Ring enhancing, central hypodense area (necrosis)—also seen with abscesses, metastases, evolving infarcts

• Short duration of pre-operative symptoms

• Grossly, may appear somewhat discrete with variegated color but often widely infiltrative and frequently crosses midline structures ("butterfly glioma")

• Microscopic pathology
  ○ Geographic necrosis
  ○ Perinecrotic pseudopalisading
  ○ Usually areas of prominent cellularity and nuclear pleomorphism
  ○ Readily identifiable mitotic figures
  ○ Vascular or endothelial proliferation
    ▶ Proliferation and piling up of cells around vascular lumina
    ▶ Capillary and glomeruloid appearances
    ▶ Some cells participating in the vascular proliferation are Factor VIII negative

    ▶ Polymorphous cell proliferation— smooth muscle cells, pericytes, adventitia, endothelial cells
    ▶ Also seen in anaplastic oligodendrogliomas, anaplastic ependymoma, pilocytic astrocytoma, abscess
  ○ A number of histologic variants exist—small cell, metaplastic, epithelioid, granular cell, spongioblastomatous, giant cell (monstrocellular sarcoma of Zulch)

• Most tumors focally GFAP positive, S-100 positive, vimentin positive; negative for cytokeratin markers (*note:* some cross-immunoreactivity with certain keratin immunostains such as AE1/3)

• Differential diagnosis
  ○ Radiation change
    ▶ Lack of perinecrotic pseudopalisading
    ▶ Microcalcifications in necrosis
    ▶ Vascular changes (hyalinized, sclerotic vessel walls)
    ▶ Bizarre cytologic atypia and cytoplasmic vacuolization
    ▶ Macrophages associated with necrosis
  ○ Metastatic carcinoma
    ▶ Discrete gross lesion
    ▶ No fibrillary background
    ▶ Collagenous stroma
    ▶ Discrete cell borders
    ▶ No perinecrotic pseudopalisading
    ▶ Generally no vascular proliferation
    ▶ Epithelial appearing cells
    ▶ Epithelial membrane antigen (EMA) and cytokeratin positive (some cytokeratin markers such as AE1/3 cross-react with gliomas), most GFAP negative

• More favorable prognosis
  ○ Young age (<45 yr)
  ○ Long duration of preoperative symptoms
  ○ Favorable neurologic condition

- ○ Presence of a substantial, better differentiated component
- ○ Extent of resection
- ○ Prominent giant-cell component (controversial)
- ○ Lower rate of cell proliferation
- Clinical course
  - ○ Without therapy: 14–16 wk
  - ○ With therapy: about 1 yr
  - ○ Chemotherapy generally not useful, treated with radiation
  - ○ Metastases
    - ▶ #1 lung
    - ▶ #2 bone

G. Multifocality in glial tumors
- GBM is most common
- 2–5%
- Increased recognition related to degree of tissue sampling
- No age difference

H. Gliosarcoma
- Feigin tumor
- Considered by many to be a GBM variant, genetic changes similar to GBM
- <2% of GBMs
- Similar presenting features, age, distribution and prognosis as GBM
- Temporal lobe most common site
- Sarcoma and GBM microscopically
- Increased metastases—sarcoma part
- Sarcoma may be fibrosarcoma, malignant fibrous histiocytoma (MFH); rarely chondrosarcoma, rhabdomyosarcoma, or angiosarcoma
- In some tumors, identical genetic abnormalities present in both components of the tumor, supporting the notion that these components arise from a single cell of origin

I. Gliomatosis cerebri
- Diffusely infiltrative glioma (WHO grade III)
- Peak incidence age 40-50 yr
- Diffuse, symmetric enlargement of brain, loss of normal architectural landmarks
- Altered behavior and mentation, seizures, headaches, focal deficits
- Most diagnosed postmortem (difficult to diagnose on biopsy alone)
- Microscopic pathology
  - ○ Undifferentiated cells with foci of higher-grade tumor
  - ○ Peripheral margin cells are elongated and slender
  - ○ Mitotic activity variable
  - ○ GFAP positive
  - ○ Secondary structures of Sherer
- Cell of origin not known
- Poor prognosis

J. Pilocytic astrocytoma
- WHO grade I
- Most common glioma in children, associated with neurofibromatosis type I
- Locations—cerebellum, wall third ventricle, optic nerve, temporal lobe, thalamus, basal ganglia
- Presentation most commonly includes focal neurological deficits or increased intracranial pressure symptoms
- Discrete cystic mass; radiographically a cystic tumor with enhancing mural nodule(s)
- Microscopic pathology
  - ○ Nuclear pleomorphism—a degenerative change
  - ○ Mitoses rare
  - ○ Vascular proliferation and sclerosis
  - ○ Biphasic appearance
    - ▶ Microcystic, loose and reticular areas
    - ▶ Compact areas with more spindled cells
    - ▶ Granular eosinophilic bodies or cells with protein drops, seen in loose areas
    - ▶ Rosenthal fibers more common in compact areas
  - ○ Microcysts
  - ○ Rarely lobular without cysts
- Clinical course

- Grow slowly, low rates of cell proliferation
- Better survival with gross total or radical subtotal excision
- 5 yr survival: 85%; 10 yr survival: 79%
- Malignant transformation rare
- Infiltration of the meninges does not adversely affect prognosis.

K. Protoplasmic astrocytoma
- Young patients (males > females)
- Mixtures of protoplasmic and fibrillary cells
- Superficial
- Cysts grossly and microscopically
- Fairly well demarcated
- Short processes, fibril poor
- GFAP immunostaining variable
- Favorable prognosis?

L. Subependymal giant-cell astrocytoma
- Increased intracranial pressure (obstruction of foramina of Monro)
- Associated with tuberous sclerosis (<20 yr), can occur later in life
- Males = females
- WHO grade I
- Elevated nodule, wall of anterior lateral ventricle
- Often associated with smaller hamartomas, which have been likened to "candle drippings"
- Discrete grossly and microscopically
- Microscopic pathology
  - Giant cells with glassy eosinophilic cytoplasm
  - Smaller elongated cells in background
  - Coarsely fibrillar background
  - Rare mitoses
  - GFAP positive
- Good prognosis, low recurrence rate

M. Pleomorphic xanthoastrocytoma
- First two decades most commonly
- Seizures 1st decade of life
- WHO grade II tumor

- Origin still debated, most classify as an astrocytoma (GFAP positive); Scattered cells in tumor stain with neuronal markers, recently described association with cortical dysplasia implies possible maldevelopmental origin
- Temporal or parietal lobes
- Cystic with mural nodule(s) configuration
- Nodules—superficial, in contact with leptomeninges
- Abrupt interface with adjacent parenchyma
- Microscopic pathology
  - Densely cellular central areas
  - Periphery less cellular
  - Pleomorphic cells
  - Lipidization of astrocytes
  - Perivascular lymphocytes
  - Reticulin rich
  - Necrosis absent
  - Mitoses rare, generally low rates of cell proliferation
  - Rare anaplastic lesions with increased mitoses and necrosis exist
  - GBM in differential diagnosis—necrosis, mitoses, older age, vascular proliferation, reticulin poor
- Generally favorable prognosis
- Rare anaplastic change (increased mitoses and necrosis), malignant transformation or recurrence in 10–25%

N. Brain stem glioma
- Childhood, rarely adults
- Generally unresectable
- Cranial nerve palsies, long tract signs, gait disturbances, vomiting, and cerebellar dysfunction
- Grossly may present as enlargement of brain stem without a discrete mass
- Bilateral or unilateral
- May be lobulated mass, may encircle basilar artery
- Microscopic pathology
  - Fasciculated and elongated cells

  ○ May see anaplastic astrocytoma or GBM

  ○ Most fibrillary, diffuse astrocytomas

  ○ Some pilocytic (10–15%)—better circumscribed, less infiltrative

O. Optic nerve glioma

- 1st decade
- Neurofibromatosis type I associated—bilateral
- Adults—anterior optic pathway, aggressive
- Visual loss
- Grow within optic sheath—enlarged optic nerve
- Fusiform enlargement
- Posterior lesion—exophytic suprasellar chiasmal mass
- Microscopic pathology
  - Two patterns
    - ▶ Lacy, low cellularity, lacking polarity, cystic foci with mucoid material
    - ▶ Fibrillated cells in bundles delineated by nerve septae
  - Rosenthal fibers (if pilocytic)
  - Nuclei with little anaplasia
  - Adults—anaplastic and GBM forms
  - Rare mitoses, necrosis, endothelial proliferation
  - Evaluate margin
- Clinical course
  - Slow growing—pilocytic types in children
  - Long survival—anterior to optic chiasm
  - Optic nerve and chiasm—location, age, extent of resection important factors
  - 5% recur after total excision
  - Radiation therapy for incomplete excision

P. Nasal glioma

- Congenital anterior displacement of non-neoplastic glial tissue
- No connection to brain (encephalocele if a connection is present)
- Disfigurement, obstruction, CSF rhinorrhea, meningitis
- Disorganized mixture of neuroglia and fibrovascular tissue
- Treat by excision
- Not truly a glioma, more akin to heterotopic or ectopic neuroglial tissue
- Other sites of glial heterotopia include occipital bone, nasopharynx, scalp, subcutaneous tissue of temporal and parietal regions

Q. Astroblastoma

- Young adults
- Variable prognosis, tumors with high-grade histological features tend to behave more aggressively
- Cerebral hemispheres
- Discrete mass
- Microscopic pathology
  - Solid, elongated cells that radiate from vasculature
  - Slight or moderate nuclear pleomorphism
  - Rare mitoses
  - GFAP and S-100 positive
  - Overlap with ordinary astrocytomas

R. Desmoplastic cerebral astrocytoma of infancy

- Superficial, frequently dural based
- <1 yr of age
- Desmoplasia
- Derived from subpial astrocytes
- Frontal or parietal lobe
- Cystic
- No giant cells, no lipidization, no ganglion cells (if ganglion cells present—desmoplastic infantile ganglioglioma)
- GFAP positive
- Favorable prognosis

S. Gliofibroma

- Rare
- Tumors with malignant glial component and abundant collagen
- Generally well-circumscribed, firm mass
- Islands, cords, or single glial cells in a collagen stroma

- Behavior seems to be dictated by grade of glioma

T. Chordoid glioma

- Rare, slow growing
- Most arise in 3rd ventricle in adults
- Solid tumors composed of clusters or cords of epithelioid cells with a variably mucinous stroma
- GFAP positive
- Mitoses rare
- Stromal lymphoplasmacytic infiltrate often with numerous Russell bodies
- Tends to recur if incompletely excised

U. Ganglioglioma

- WHO grade I tumor
- May be confused with astrocytoma
- Most common in temporal lobe
- Children > adults
- Most patients present with chronic epilepsy
- Cystic tumor with calcified mural nodule
- A glioneuronal tumor; microscopically need to identify both atypical ganglionic (neuronal) cell component and a glioma component
- Atypical neurons may be binucleated
- Calcifications common
- Granular bodies
- Rare or absent mitoses
- Perivascular lymphocytes
- Associated with coexistent cortical dysplasia, possible maldevelopmental origin
- Generally good prognosis with complete excision; rare aggressive tumors reported
- Desmoplastic infantile ganglioglioma— very young patients, large size, superficial location
- Gangliocytoma—tumor composed of mature ganglion cells
- Dysplastic gangliocytoma of the cerebellum (Lhermitte-Duclos)—occurs in setting of Cowden syndrome caused by phosphatase and tensin homolog deleted on chromosome 10 (PTEN) germline mutation, hamartomatous lesion of ganglion cells

II. Oligodendroglial Neoplasms

A. Oligodendroglioma

- 5–15% of glial neoplasms
- Long history of signs and symptoms (mean 1–5 yr) prior to diagnosis
- Seizures, headaches most common symptoms; about 20% hemorrhage
- Adults > children; mean age 35–45 yr
- WHO grade II lesion
- White matter
- Frontal lobe>parietal>temporal>occipital
- Microscopic pathology
  - Sheets of cells, distinct cytoplasmic borders
  - Vacuolated "fried egg" appearance— formalin-fixation artifact
  - Central nucleus, minimal pleomorphism
  - Arcuate or "chicken wire" vascular pattern
  - Calcification—prominent at periphery, seen in 90% of cases
  - Cortical invasion
  - May see meningeal invasion with desmoplasia
  - Subpial and perineuronal arrangement of tumor cells
  - May see microcystic change
  - Rare mitoses at most
  - Occasional signet-ring cell variant (degenerative phenomenon), no clinical significance
- GFAP negative or focally positive; S-100, A2B5, and Leu-7 positive
- Cell proliferation marker labeling indices low
- Molecular genetics
  - Most frequent genetic alteration present is LOH chromosome 19q
  - Other abnormalities include LOH 1p and 4q
  - TP53 mutations relatively rare
- Generally difficult to totally resect
- Most do not survive beyond 10 yr

- Radiation therapy of debated use, more likely to be chemoresponsive
- May dedifferentiate with time

B. Anaplastic oligodendroglioma
- WHO grade III tumor
- Pleomorphic nuclei
- Mitoses, often > 5 per high-power fields
- Vascular proliferation
- Necrosis
- Increased cellularity
- Worse prognosis than low-grade tumor, median survival 3–4 yr
- Rarely can see "glioblastoma multiforme" derived from oligodendroglial tumor
- 1p and 19q chromosome deletions associated with increased likelihood of chemoresponsiveness

C. Mixed glioma
- Clinically and radiographically similar to astrocytomas and oligodendrogliomas
- Most frequently a mixture of astrocytoma and oligodendroglioma (oligoastrocytoma), 20–30% minor component
- May have anaplastic tumor components present (malignant mixed glioma)
- A subset of tumors have genetic alterations similar to oligodendroglioma
- Prognosis may be intermediate between pure oligodendroglioma and astrocytoma
- Rarely see mixtures of other glioma types (oligoependymoma and ependymoma—astrocytoma)

D. Dysembryoplastic neuroepithelial tumor
- WHO grade I tumor
- An oligodendroglioma look-alike
- Young patients, childhood, chronic epilepsy history
- Multinodular, multicystic, cortical based
- Associated with cortical dysplasia (maldevelopmental lesion)
- Mixture of predominantly oligodendroglial cells with fewer numbers of neurons and astrocytes arranged against a microcystic background, no significant cytologic atypia
- Temporal lobe most common site

- Mitoses rare, low rates of cell proliferation
- Good prognosis, potentially curable with complete excision

E. Central neurocytoma
- WHO grade II tumor
- Another oligodendroglioma look-alike
- Discrete, often partly calcified
- Intraventricular near septum pellucidum or in 3rd ventricle
- Rare examples of extraventricular neurocytoma have been reported including the papillary glioneuronal tumor and cerebellar liponeurocytoma
- Most frequent in young adults
- Uniform nuclei with speckled chromatin
- Perivascular pattern, pseudorosettes
- Fibrillary background
- May be focally calcified
- Mitoses generally rare
- Generally GFAP negative, synaptophysin positive
- Dense core granules on electron microscopy (evidence of neuronal differentiation)
- Surgical cure may be possible with complete excision

III. Ependymal Neoplasms
A. Rosettes
- True rosettes (tumor cells themselves form a lumen)
  ○ Flexner Wintersteiner
    ▶ Small lumen
    ▶ Cuboidal lining
    ▶ Retinoblastoma
  ○ Ependymal
    ▶ Ependymal lining
    ▶ Ciliary attachment (blepharoplast)
    ▶ Cilia in 9 : 1 orientation
    ▶ Canal/channel with long lumen
- Pseudorosettes (tumor cells arrange themselves around something)
  ○ Perivascular
    ▶ Uniformly arranged cells
    ▶ Vessel center

- ○ Homer Wright
  - ▶ Fibrillary core
  - ▶ Neuroblastic differentiation
  - ▶ Primitive neuroectodermal tumor (PNET)

B. Ependymoma
- WHO grade II tumor
- 5–10% of tumors, children
- 1–2% of brain tumors, adult
- Any ventricle (especially 4th) and spinal cord (intramedullary)
- 71% infratentorial
- Obstruction of CSF-related signs and symptoms at presentation
- Grossly: soft lobular, discrete mass, well demarcated
- Microscopic pathology
  - ○ Extreme fibrillarity
  - ○ Nuclei round to oval, "carrot-shaped"
  - ○ Dense nuclear chromatin
  - ○ Slight nuclear pleomorphism
  - ○ Infrequent mitoses
  - ○ Perivascular pseudorosettes
  - ○ True ependymal rosettes
  - ○ Blepharoplasts—intracytoplasmic, basal bodies of cilia, best seen ultrastructurally
  - ○ Variants: papillary, clear cell, tanycytic, melanotic, lipomatous, giant cell, signet-ring cell; no difference in prognosis associated with these variants
  - ○ May see heavy calcification/ossification/cartilage
- GFAP and EMA positive
- Low cell proliferation labeling indices
- Clinical course
  - ○ Better prognosis in adults, supratentorial tumors, gross total resection
  - ○ Radiation to CNS axis
  - ○ Grade is not as important as location and extent of resection
  - ○ Better differentiated lesions do better
  - ○ Spinal better than intracranial tumors

C. Anaplastic ependymoma
- WHO grade III tumor
- Rare
- Precise histologic criteria to distinguish from ordinary ependymoma is not well defined
- Increased mitoses
- Nuclear and cellular pleomorphism
- Hypercellularity
- Endothelial proliferation
- Focal necrosis frequent

D. Subependymoma
- WHO grade I tumor
- Adults; males > females
- Asymptomatic, most cases are an incidental finding at autopsy
- Small, usually <0.5 cm
- Nodular mass; soft, tan, solid
- Septum pellucidum, floor or lateral recess of the 4th ventricle
- Microscopic pathology
  - ○ "Islands of blue (nuclei) in a sea of pink (fibrillary background)"
  - ○ Nuclei-like ependymoma
  - ○ Mitoses rare, low cell proliferation marker indices
  - ○ Calcification common, microcystic change common
  - ○ GFAP positive
  - ○ No rosettes or pseudorosettes
  - ○ Microcystic change common
- Excellent prognosis, surgical removal usually curative
- More likely to recur if larger, hard to resect, mixed with true ependymoma

E. Myxopapillary ependymoma
- WHO grade I tumor
- Males > females
- Average age of diagnosis: 30–40 yr
- Lower back pain history
- Slow growing
- May be locally infiltrative, hemorrhagic, or lobular
- 25% encapsulated

- Filum terminale
- Rarely subcutaneous sacrococcygeal region
- Microscopic pathology
  - Mucoid stroma, mucicarmine, and alcian blue positive
  - Intracellular mucin
  - Recapitulate normal filum terminale
  - Papillary appearance with central vessel
  - GFAP positive
  - Some atypia and rare mitoses
- Clinical course
  - Recurrence 10–15%
  - Good prognosis
  - Radiation therapy (if not completely excised)
  - Mean survival 19 yr after total excision in one large series

IV. Dural-Based Tumors

   A. Meningioma

- 13–26% of primary intracranial tumors, incidence 6/100,000
- Associated with neurofibromatosis type II
- Any age, most common in middle-aged and elderly
- Females > males
- Associated with breast carcinoma
- May express progesterone > estrogen receptors
- Most arise proximal to meninges from arachnoidal cap cells; falx cerebri is single most common site of origin
- Rarely arise in unusual sites such as intraventricular region, head and neck region, or lung
- Most are slow growing and present with signs and symptoms related to compression of adjacent structures
- Grossly, most are well circumscribed; compress adjacent parenchyma
- May invade skull and produce hyperostosis
- Gross appearance may be variable, depending on histologic type

- A variety of benign histologic subtypes defined (WHO grade I tumors)
  - Meningothelial (syncytial) cells arranged in lobules divided by collagenous septae, whorling of cells around vessels or psammoma bodies (calcifications), eosinophilic cytoplasmic protrusions into the nuclei prominent (nuclear pseudoinclusions)
  - Fibrous (fibroblastic)—spindle cells with abundant collagen or reticulin between cells
  - Transitional (mixed)—features between meningothelial and fibrous types
  - Psammomatous—abundant calcifications
  - Angiomatous—marked by prominent vasculature, not to be confused with hemangiopericytoma or hemangioblastoma
  - Microcystic—loose, mucinous background
  - Secretory (pseudopsammomatous)—formation of intracellular lumina containing PAS positive, eosinophilic material
  - Lymphoplasmacyte rich—marked by extensive chronic inflammation
  - Metaplastic—demonstrates mesenchymal differentiation (bone, cartilage, fat)
- Marked by low rate of cell proliferation
- Immunohistochemistry: most EMA positive and vimentin positive; variable positivity with S-100 protein and cytokeratins
- Electron microscopy shows prominent interdigitated cell processes and desmosomal junctions
- May be induced by prior radiation
- Most common cytogenetic abnormality is deletion of chromosome 22; other less frequent abnormalities are deletion/loss on 1p, 6q, 9q, 10q, 14q, 17p, and 18q
- Potentially curable with gross total resection, a subset recurs over time

   B. Atypical and malignant meningiomas

- Four histologic subtypes associated with more aggressive behavior
  - Chordoid—areas similar to chordoma

with trabeculae of eosinophilic and vacuolated cells in a myxoid background, WHO grade II tumor

  - Clear cell—cells with clear, glycogen-rich cytoplasm, WHO grade II tumor

  - Papillary—perivascular pseudopapillary pattern, WHO grade III tumor

  - Rhabdoid—rhabdoid-like cells with eccentric nuclei, prominent nucleoli and cytoplasmic inclusions of intermediate filaments, WHO grade III

- Atypical meningioma marked by increased mitoses (4 or more mitotic figures/10 high power fields or 0.16 mm^2) or 3 or more of the following features: increased cellularity, small cells, prominent nucleoli, sheet-like patternless growth pattern, and foci of necrosis; WHO grade II tumor, more common in males; 4.7–7.2% of meningiomas, more likely to recur than grade I tumors.

- Malignant (anaplastic meningioma) marked by histological features of frank malignancy, 20 or more mitotic figures per 10 high power fields (0.16 mm^2), brain invasion (rarely seen in lower-grade lesions), or metastases; WHO grade III tumor, median survival less than 2 yr

C. Mesenchymal, nonmeningothelial tumors

- Includes a variety of benign and malignant lesions, histologically resembling their extra CNS counterparts

- Benign lesions one can see include lipoma (adipose), angiolipoma (adipose and prominent vasculature), hibernoma (brown fat), fibromatosis, solitary fibrous tumor (CD34 positive), benign fibrous histiocytoma (fibrous xanthoma), leiomyoma (smooth muscle, AIDS associated), rhabdomyoma (striated muscle), chondroma (cartilage), osteoma (bone), osteochondroma (bone), hemangioma (capillary or cavernous) and epithelioid hemangioendothelioma

- Malignant lesions one can encounter include a variety of sarcomas (liposarcoma, fibrosarcoma, malignant fibrous histiocytoma, leiomyosarcoma, rhabdomyosarcoma, osteosarcoma, chondrosarcoma, angiosarcoma, and Kaposi's sarcoma)

- Chordoma

  - Derived from notochordal tissue remnants (ecchordosis physaliphora)

  - Most arise in spheno-occipital region or clivus and sacrococcygeal region

  - Bone-based tumors, lobulated, may appear grossly mucoid

  - May contain cartilage (chondroid chordoma)

  - Microscopically consists of epithelioid cells arrayed against a mucoid matrix

  - Some cells with marked vacuolation (physaliphorous or bubble cells)

  - Immunoreactive for vimentin, cytokeratin, EMA, S-100 protein

  - Locally recur, occasionally metastasize

  - Gross total resection and young age (<40 yr) do better

D. Hemangiopericytoma

- Relatively rare sarcoma of CNS

- Men > women

- Mean age of diagnosis 40–50 yr

- May cause lytic destruction of adjacent bone, no hyperostosis

- Grossly a solid, well-demarcated mass, tends to bleed during removal

- WHO grade II or III tumors

- Histologically, highly cellular

- Cells randomly oriented

- Numerous staghorn contoured vessels

- Reticulin rich

- Calcification/psammoma bodies not seen

- Variably see mitotic figures, necrosis

- Immunohistochemistry: most stain with vimentin, CD34; EMA negative

- May be pericytic in origin

- Decreased survival has been associated with increased mitosis (5 or more mitotic figures/10 high-power fields), high cellularity, nuclear pleomorphism, hemorrhage and necrosis

- Treated by surgery and radiation, most eventually recur, 60–70% eventually metastasize

E. Melanocytic lesions

- Melanocytoma

- ○ 0.06–0.1% of brain tumors
- ○ Any age, females > males
- ○ Monomorphic spindled or epithelioid cells rich in melanin
- ○ Mitotic activity low, minimal necrosis
- ○ May recur locally
- Diffuse melanocytosis
  - ○ Children
  - ○ Leptomeningeal based proliferation of nevoid cells
  - ○ Associated with neurocutaneous melanosis syndrome
  - ○ Poor prognosis
- Primary meningeal melanoma
  - ○ Very rare
  - ○ Marked by cytologic atypia, high mitotic counts, necrosis, hemorrhage
  - ○ Poor prognosis

F. Hemangioblastoma
- May not necessarily be dural based
- Young adults
- Cerebellum most common site, less commonly brain stem and spinal cord
- Cyst with enhancing mural nodule appearance radiographically
- Associated with von Hippel-Lindau disease (chromosome 3p)
- Associated with secondary polycythemia vera (produces erythropoietin)
- Uncertain histogenesis
- WHO grade I tumor
- Histologically marked by rich capillary network and intermixed vacuolated stromal cells
- May show cystic changes and nuclear pleomorphism
- Mitoses and necrosis not prominent
- EMA negative by immunohistochemistry (to distinguish from EMA-positive metastatic renal cell carcinoma in von Hippel-Lindau setting)
- Prognosis generally good

V. Choroid Plexus Tumors
A. Choroid plexus papilloma
- Most present in the 1st two decades of life
- Lateral ventricle in children
- 4th ventricle more common in adults
- Presentation often related to CSF obstruction symptoms
- Circumscribed, papillary mass
- WHO grade I tumor
- Pathologically marked by a hyperplasia of bland epithelial-type cells on collagen–vascular cores
- Not much atypia, mitotic activity, necrosis, or brain invasion
- May rarely contain metaplastic elements (bone, cartilage) or demonstrate oncocytic change or mucinous degeneration
- Most stain with antibodies to cytokeratins, vimentin, S-100 protein; up to half stain focally with GFAP
- Can seed cells in the CSF space
- Low rates of cell proliferation
- Associated with SV40 DNA sequences
- Associated with LiFraumeni syndrome
- Potentially curable by surgery with 5-yr survival rate of up to 100%
- Occasional tumors with worrisome histology (not enough to call carcinoma) designated as atypical choroid plexus papilloma

B. Choroid plexus carcinoma
- About 80% arise in children
- Same locations as papilloma
- WHO grade III tumor
- Grossly invasive, solid, and necrotic
- Histologically demonstrates features of frank malignancy—atypia, increased mitoses, solid areas, necrosis, and brain invasion
- High rates of cell proliferation
- 5-yr survival rate of about 40%

VI. Embryonal Tumors
A. Myoepithelioma
- Rare, children 6 mo–5 yr
- Most commonly arise in periventricular region in cerebral hemispheres

- Often large in size and well circumscribed at presentation
- WHO grade IV tumor
- Mimics histologically the embryonic neural tube
- Papillary, tubular, or trabecular arrangements of neuroepithelial cells which may demonstrate neural, glial, or mesenchymal differentiation
- Mitoses abundant, necrosis common
- Generally poor prognosis, rapidly growing, radiation may provide some benefit

B. Ependymoblastoma
- Rare, young children
- Most supratentorial, large in size
- WHO grade IV tumor
- Dense cellularity
- Multilayered rosettes, outer cells of rosettes merge with adjacent undifferentiated embryonal tumor
- Prominent mitoses
- Grow rapidly, disseminate readily, poor prognosis

C. Medulloblastoma
- Peak in 1st decade, 70% occur in children <16 yr
- Males > females
- Most arise in vermis and project into 4th ventricle
- Clinical presentation most commonly ataxia, gait disturbance, headache, vomiting
- WHO grade IV tumor
- Typical histopathology marked by densely packed cells with high nuclear-to-cytoplasmic ratio
- Homer Wright pseudorosettes <40% of cases
- Mitoses frequent, apoptosis frequent
- Necrosis common
- Desmoplastic variant marked by nodular, reticulin-free zones (pale islands) surrounded by more densely cellular areas (reticulin rich)
- Nodular variant marked by intranodular nuclear uniformity, cell streaming, neurocytic-like cells

- Large cell variant marked by large, pleomorphic cells with prominent nucleoli
- Medullomyoblastoma marked by focal myogenic differentiation
- Melanotic medulloblastoma marked by melanotic cells, often epithelial in appearance and forming tubules
- Many stain with synaptophysin antibody; subset GFAP positive
- Cytogenetics: about half with isochromosome 17q, loss of part of 17p in 30–45%, loss on 1q and 10q in 20–40%
- 5-yr survival—50–70%
- Poor prognosis associated with young age (<3 yr), metastasis at presentation, subtotal resection, large cell variant, melanotic variant

D. Cerebral neuroblastoma
- AKA: Supratentorial primitive neuroectodermal tumor (PNET)
- Most arise in 1st decade
- Presentation with seizures, disturbances of consciousness, focal motor deficits
- WHO grade IV tumor
- Histologically similar in appearance to medulloblastoma
- More than half calcified
- May contain areas with terminally differentiated cells (ganglion cells)—ganglioneuroblastoma
- 5-yr survival (30–40%)

E. Atypical teratoid/rhabdoid tumor
- Most arise in infants or children
- Slightly more common in males
- About half arise in posterior fossa
- About a third present with metastases throughout CSF axis
- WHO grade IV tumor
- Histologically marked by rhabdoid cells with eosinophilic cytoplasm, eccentric nucleus, prominent nucleolus
- Cytoplasmic "pink body"—corresponds to collections of intermediate filaments
- May contain a small cell embryonal component or mesenchymal component
- Mitoses and necrosis common
- Rhabdoid cells by immunohistochemistry

express EMA and vimentin; variably express neurofilament protein, GFAP, smooth-muscle actin and cytokeratin immunoreactivity

- 90% demonstrate monosomy or deletion on chromosome 22
- Most patients die within 1 yr of diagnosis

VII. Peripheral Nerve Tumors

   A. Schwannoma

- AKA: neurilemmoma, neurinoma, acoustic neuroma
- Arises from peripheral nerve
- 8% of intracranial and 29% of primary spinal cord tumors
- Associated with neurofibromatosis type I
- Any age, peak 4th–6th decades
- WHO grade I lesion
- Many are encapsulated, globoid masses
- Composed microscopically of spindled cells with alternating areas of compact cells (Antoni A pattern) and less cellular looser regions (Antoni B pattern)
- Cell nuclei with tapered ends
- May demonstrate nuclear pleomorphism (ancient change)
- May show nuclear palisading Verocay bodies
- May contain lipid-like cells or undergo cystic degeneration
- Frequently has thickened vessel walls
- Cellular schwannoma variant–hypercellular, mostly Antoni A pattern
- Melanotic schwannoma–grossly and microscopically pigmented (melanin), about 50% of tumors with psammoma bodies associated with Carney complex (autosomal dominant disorder marked by cardiac myxomas, endocrine abnormalities and pigmented skin lesions), about 10% follow a malignant course
- Plexiform schwannoma—associated with neurofibromatosis type II
- Immunohistochemistry—strong and diffuse staining with S-100 protein
- Slow growing, benign tumors

   B. Neurofibroma

- Any age
- Painful masses
- Associated with neurofibromatosis type I
- WHO grade I tumor
- Grossly may present as a cutaneous nodule or as a diffuse lesion; plexiform tumors are multinodular "bag of worms"
- Histologically composed of an admixture of Schwann cells, perineurial-like cells and fibroblasts in a mucoid/loose matrix
- Mitoses rare, atypia usually not prominent, cellularity typically low
- May contain tactile-like structures (Wagner-Meissner-like corpuscles)
- Scattered S-100 positivity
- Plexiform tumors and those arising in large nerves may give rise to malignant peripheral nerve sheath tumors (MPNST)
  - AKA: neurogenic sarcoma, neurofibrosarcoma, malignant schwannoma
  - About half of MPNST arise in neurofibromatosis I
  - Histologically marked by hypercellularity, necrosis, increased mitoses
  - Frequently invasive
  - Variant types include epithelioid, glandular, and Triton tumor (rhabdomyosarcomatous differentiation)
  - Poor prognosis, 5-yr survival about 35%

   C. Perineurioma

- Rare benign tumor comprised of perineurial cells
- Presents in adolescence or young adults
- Progressive muscle weakness (intraneural tumors) and mass effect (soft tissue tumors)
- Intraneural tumors present with segmental nerve enlargement
- Microscopically see proliferating perineurial cells in endoneurium around nerve fibers (pseudo-onion bulbs)
- Soft-tissue tumors comprised of spindled, wavy cells
- EMA positive by immunohistochemistry
- Benign clinical course

D. Neuromas

- Traumatic or amputation neuroma marked by fibrosis and disorderly arrangement of nerve twigs/fibers

- Morton's neuroma thickening and degeneration of interdigital nerve of foot, presents with pain, histologically digital artery wall thickened ± occluded with fibrosis of nerve

VIII. Hematopoietic Tumors

A. Lymphoma

- Increasing incidence in recent years

- Associated with AIDS

- All ages, peak 6th–7th decades in immunocompetent persons

- Males > females

- 60% supratentorial

- 25–50% multiple (60–85% in AIDS and posttransplant patients)

- Most present with focal neurological deficits or neuropsychiatric symptoms

- CSF cytology pleocytosis observed in 35–60% of patients, cytology diagnostic in 5–30% of primary CNS lymphomas, and 70–95% of metastatic lymphomas (which tend to be leptomeningeal based)

- Histologically marked by angiocentric, atypical lymphoid cell infiltrate

- Most primary CNS lymphomas are non Hodgkin's lymphomas, diffuse large cell type, B-cell immunophenotype (CD20, CD79a positive)

- Tumor cells may be admixed with variable numbers of smaller tumor infiltrating lymphocytes (T-cells)

- About 2% are T-cell lymphomas

- Other rare lymphoma types to involve CNS include angiotropic large cell lymphoma or intravascular lymphoma (cells are confined primarily to vascular lumens, large B-cells), Hodgkin's lymphoma (Reed Sternberg cells—CD30 and CD15 positive) and mucosa-associated lymphoid tissue (MALT) lymphoma of dura (low-grade B-cell lymphoma; CD20 and CD79a positive; CD5, CD10, and CD23 negative)

- Epstein-Barr virus genome present in most tumors in immunocompromised patients

- Gene rearrangement studies by polymerase chain reaction may help in identifying tumors where the number of cells present is low

- Favorable prognosis in patients with single lesion, absence of meningeal or periventricular tumor, immunocompetent, age <60 yr, and preoperative Karnofsky score >70

- 85% response rate, median survival 17–45 mo

- Very steroid-responsive initially

B. Histiocytic Tumors

- Langerhan's cell histiocytosis

  o Children

  o Multifocal involvement of bone and brain (Hand-Schüller-Christian disease) or skin, nodes, viscera, and rarely CNS (Letterer-Siwe disease)

  o Grossly appear as yellow or white dural nodules or granular parenchymal infiltrate

  o Granulomatous infiltrates marked by Langerhan's cell histiocytes (eccentric nuclei, linear grooved nucleus, inconspicuous nucleoli, CD1a positive, Birbeck granules by electron microscopy—34-nm-wide rod-shaped or tennis-racket-shaped intracytoplasmic pentalaminar structures), lymphocytes, plasma cells and eosinophils

  o Overall survival 88% at 5 yr

- Non-Langerhans cell histiocytosis

  o Macrophage differentiation, absence of features of dendritic Langerhans cell

  o Rosai-Dorfman disease—adults, dural based, sheets or nodules of histiocytes (CD1a negative, CD11c positive, CD68 positive)

  o Erdheim-Chester disease—adults, lipid-laden macrophages (CD1a negative, CD68 positive, S-100 protein negative) and multinucleated Touton giant cells

  o Hemophagocytic lymphohistiocytosis—autosomal recessive, infants; infiltrates of lymphocytes and macrophages with hemophagocytosis and variable necrosis

IX. Cysts

    A. Colloid Cyst

- Third ventricle
- Young to middle-aged adults
- Headaches, transient paralysis of lower extremities, incontinence, personality changes
- Histologically marked by a single layer of columnar epithelial cells, may contain goblet and ciliated cells
- Amorphous, brightly eosinophilic cyst fluid
- May see filamentous-like masses of nucleoprotein
- Positive for EMA and cytokeratin markers by immunohistochemistry

    B. Rathke's cleft cyst

- Intrasellar or suprasellar
- Often incidental finding, larger ones may be symptomatic causing visual disturbances or abnormalities of hypothalamic pituitary function
- Histologically lined by ciliated columnar epithelium, may see squamous metaplasia

    C. Endodermal cyst

- Any age, many are intraspinal
- AKA: enterogenous, neurenteric, enterogenic cysts
- Histologically consists of cuboidal to columnar epithelium lying on fibrovascular capsule

    D. Ependymal cyst—intraparenchymal or periventricular cyst lined by ependymal type cells

    E. Choroid plexus cyst—epithelial-lined cyst of the choroid plexus

    F. Arachnoid cyst

- Subarachnoid space in the temporal lobe region is favored site
- Delicate, translucent wall filled with clear fluid
- EMA positive by immunohistochemistry

    G. Synovial cysts of spine

- AKA: ganglion cyst
- Intradural, extramedullary lesions associated with degenerative joint disease
- Fibrous capsule containing gelatinous fluid, no epithelial lining

    H. Dermoid and epidermoid cysts

- Arise from embryologically misplaced epithelial cells either in meninges, ventricles, or brain parenchyma
- Epidermoid: cerebellopontine angle most common site, may occur in other sites (i.e., suprasellar)
- Dermoid: posterior fossa, midline lesions, 4th ventricle
- Macroscopic pathology
  - Epidermoid: smooth, translucent cyst, when open has flaky contents
  - Dermoid: thicker capsule with pilosebaceous contents
- Microscopic pathology
  - Epidermoid: keratin debris, keratohyaline granules, and delicate epithelial lining
  - Dermoid: epithelial-lined cyst with sweat and sebaceous glands
  - Cysts can rupture and elicit a foreign-body giant-cell reaction to their contents

X. Miscellaneous Tumors

    A. Paraganglioma

- Most present as spinal intradural tumors in the cauda equina region
- Intracranial tumors usually represent extensions of jugulotympanic tumors
- Mean age 40–50 yr, males > females
- Often present with lower back pain
- WHO grade I tumor
- Composed of chief cells arranged in nests or lobules (zellballen) surrounded by a single layer of sustentacular cells
- May encounter mild pleomorphism, occasional mitotic figures, and rarely foci of hemorrhagic necrosis
- Chief cells stain with synaptophysin, chromogranin, and neurofilament proteins
- Sustentacular cells stain with S-100 protein
- Most in cauda equina are slow growing and potentially curable by total excision

- Cannot predict behavior of tumor based on histology

B. Pineocytoma

- Most common in adolescence and adulthood
- Less prone than pineoblastoma to seed the CSF
- Survival information scanty
- Microscopic pathology
  - Lobular, small cells
  - Largely hypocellular zones of fibrillarity that resemble Homer-Wright rosettes (pineocytomatous rosettes)
  - Fibrillary zones have neural nature (synaptophysin, neuron-specific enolase, and neurofilament protein positive)

C. Germ cell neoplasms

- Occur along the midline, most commonly suprasellar region and pineal
- Suprasellar tumors equally divided among males and females, pineal tumors with male predominance
- Most occur in 1st three decades
- Common signs and symptoms: headache, papilledema, mental status changes, gaze palsies, precocious puberty
- Diffuse dissemination occasionally seen
- Histologically the same as germ cell tumors of the ovary or testis (germinoma, teratoma, yolk sac tumor, embryonal carcinoma, choriocarcinoma)
- Germinoma is the most common CNS germ cell tumor

D. Craniopharyngioma

- Rare tumors of the sellar region
  - Two peaks: 1st two decades and the 6th–7th decades
  - Local recurrence
  - Presents with disturbances in the hypothalamic–pituitary axis, visual symptoms, CSF symptoms (obstruction)
  - May originate from squamous cells at the base of the infundibular stalk
- Macroscopic pathology
  - Fill suprasellar region, displace or attach to cranial nerves and vessels
  - Cut section: necrotic debris, calcium, "cystic oil" often with cholesterol
  - Spillage of the oil may result in chemical meningitis
- Microscopic pathology
  - Cells form compact masses or line cysts
  - Assume an adamantinomatous pattern: peripheral palisading of epithelial cells admixed with a loose "stellate reticulum"
  - Keratin-containing cells
  - Histiocytes, calcium, and cholesterol clefts seen
  - Surrounding brain has intense gliosis and Rosenthal fiber formation

E. Pituitary adenoma

- About 10–20% of all intracranial neoplasms
- Most common in adults
- Women most often affected
- Seen incidentally in approximately 25% of autopsies
- Microadenoma <1 cm in diameter
- Symptoms: related to endocrine dysfunction or visual disturbance
- Most common secreting adenoma—prolactinoma
- Microscopic pathology
  - Heterogeneous histologic appearance
  - Patterned sheets of uniform cells with a delicate vascular network
  - Nuclei are round and have a delicate chromatin pattern
  - Cells often have granular cytoplasm
  - Lacks the normal acinar or lobular pattern of the pituitary
  - Monotonous cell types
  - Immunohistochemical staining for pituitary hormones will identify the secretory products
- Rare examples of pituitary carcinoma (defined by noncontiguous spread)
- Apoplexy—sudden enlargement of adenoma related to infarct/hemorrhage

F. Metastatic disease

- Common

- Typically found in patients 5th–7th decades

- Often multiple, may be ring-enhancing lesions radiographically

- Associated with prominent edema

- Most common in descending order of incidence: lung, breast, melanoma, renal cell, gastrointestinal tumors

- Common in all areas of brain

- 70% of patients have more than one metastasis

- Distributed in arterial watershed zones

- Associated with edema, which may be out of proportion to tumor size

- Frequently at the gray–white junction

- Discrete, sharply demarcated from adjacent brain grossly

- Microscopic pathology

  o Distinctive nuclear characteristics, resembling the primary tumor

  o Vascular proliferation uncommon

  o Immunohistochemical staining with cytokeratins often positive and distinctive

  o Cells often cohesive

G. Lipoma

- Usually midline: corpus callosum, 3rd ventricular region, cerebellopontine (CP) angle, quadrigeminal area

- May be associated with developmental abnormalities (i.e., agenesis of the corpus callosum)

- Usually incidental autopsy findings; rarely associated with seizures

- Color (yellow) is essential feature and calcification may be seen peripherally

- Composed of mature fat and blood vessels

XI. Common Tumors by Location

A. Cerebral hemisphere

- Astrocytoma (diffuse, fibrillary type)

- Oligodendroglioma

- Metastatic carcinoma

- Glioneuronal tumors

- Ependymoma (near ventricle)

- Meningioma/sarcoma (dural based)

- Lymphoma

- Neuroblastoma

B. Corpus callosum

- Astrocytoma

- Oligodendroglioma

- Lipoma

C. Lateral ventricle

- Ependymoma

- Choroid plexus papilloma

- Subependymoma

- Central neurocytoma

D. Third ventricle

- Ependymoma

- Colloid cyst

- Pilocytic astrocytoma (adjacent)

E. Fourth ventricle

- Ependymoma

- Choroid plexus papilloma

- Meningioma

F. Optic nerve/chiasm

- Astrocytoma

- Meningioma

G. Pituitary/sella

- Adenoma

- Craniopharyngioma

- Germ cell tumor

- Meningioma

- Rathke's cleft cyst

H. Cerebellum

- Hemangioblastoma

- Medulloblastoma

- Astrocytoma

- Metastasis

- Dermoid cyst

I. Pineal gland

- Germ cell tumor (especially germinoma)

- Pineocytoma

- Pineoblastoma

J. Cerebellopontine angle

- Schwannoma

- Meningioma

- Epidermoid cyst
- Ependymoma
- Choroid plexus papilloma

K. Brain stem
  - Astrocytoma—diffuse, fibrillary type versus pilocytic

L. Spinal cord
  - Intramedullary
    - Ependymoma
    - Astrocytoma

- Intradural, extramedullary
  - Schwannoma
  - Meningioma
  - Myxopapillary ependymoma
  - Paraganglioma
  - Chordoma
- Extradural
  - Metastasis
  - Lymphoma
  - Myeloma

4 Trauma

I. Herniation Syndromes

A. General information

- Herniation is a significant cause of CNS morbidity and mortality.

- Alterations in intracranial dynamics causing increased intracranial pressure (ICP) operate by a variety of mechanisms

  ○ Rapid growth, rather than size of growth often the more critical factor

  ○ Location of the mass relative to CSF and venous outflow is important

  ○ Increased ICP also related to tissue edema

B. Generalized brain swelling (edema)—increase in brain volume because of increased tissue water content

- Gyri flattened

- Narrow sulci

- Prominent pacchionian granulations

- In chronic cases, bony erosion may result

- Increased brain weight

- Obstruction of subarachnoid space and decreased ventricular size.

- May be associated with congestive brain swelling—increase in cerebral blood volume in capillary and postcapillary beds

C. Types of cerebral edema

- Vasogenic

  ○ Result of blood-brain barrier breakdown

  ○ Around tumors or trauma, diffuse in white matter

  ○ Enlarged extracellular spaces with perivascular astrocyte foot process swelling

- Cytotoxic

  ○ Result of impairment of cell Na^+-K^+ membrane pump

  ○ Intracellular swelling mainly in gray matter

  ○ Hypoxia most common cause

  ○ No enlargement of extracellular spaces

D. Lateral transtentorial herniation

- AKA: parahippocampal/uncal herniation

- Usually occurs with lateral supratentorial masses

- Earliest change is displacement of the uncus and parahippocampal gyrus beneath the tentorial notch

  ○ Eventually hemorrhagic necrosis occurs

  ○ Herniating tissue alters the relationship of structures to the tentorium

  ○ Kernohan's notch—damage to the contralateral cerebral peduncle

  ○ Compression of the ispilateral 3rd nerve

  ○ Posterior cerebral artery is trapped by the parahippocampal gyrus and the ipsilateral cerebral peduncle, leading to infarction in the calcarine cortex

  ○ Midline brain stem hemorrhage, Duret hemorrhage

E. Central herniation

- Occurs with parenchymal lesions in the frontal and parietal lobes

- Extracerebral lesions near the vertex may also be responsible
- Downward displacement of the hemispheres results in herniation of the thalamus and midbrain
  - Compression of the anterior choroidal artery with subsequent infarction of the globus pallidus and optic tract

F. Subfalcial herniation

- AKA: cingulate or supracallosal herniation
- Usually associated with mass lesions in the anterior portion of the cerebrum (frontal or parietal lobe)
- Displacement of the cingulate gyrus under the falx cerebri
- Anterior cerebral artery may be displaced with resultant infarction

G. Tonsillar herniation

- Cerebellar tonsils are displaced downward into the foramen magnum
- Tonsillar tips are elongated and flattened against the medulla
- Prolonged tonsillar compression leads to hemorrhagic necrosis of the tonsils

H. Upward herniation

- Result of an expanding posterior fossa lesion
- Upward protrusion of the cerebellum through the tentorial notch with grooving of the anterior vermis and the lateral lobes
  - May cause compression of the superior cerebellar artery with infarction
  - May displace the overlying vein of Galen

I. External herniation

- Displacement of brain tissue through a defect in skull (often caused by trauma or surgery)
- Hemorrhagic infarct at edge of herniated tissue

II. Traumatic Hemorrhage

A. Epidural hematoma

- Commonly seen post-trauma, occurs in about 3% of significant head injuries
- Most are frontal or temporal and associated with a laceration of one of the meningeal arteries, most commonly the middle menin-

geal artery; secondary to a fracture (in 80–85%)

- In children, may be the result of impact alone without skull fracture
- Amount of bleeding results from a variety of factors
  - Adherence of the dura to the inner table of the skull
  - Depth of the meningeal arterial groove
  - Relationship of the fracture to the vessels
- One-third of patients with epidural hematoma have other traumatic lesions
- Epidural hematomas may deform the underlying brain with subsequent mass effect
- Majority are acute and potentially lethal if not evacuated

B. Subdural hematoma

- More common than epidural hematoma; may produce symptoms referable to mass effect or may present with fluctuating neurologic signs and headache
- Result of tearing of bridging veins which transverse through the subarachnoid space
- Acute subdural hemorrhage associated with skull fracture (50%) and diffuse axonal injury; high mortality (40–60%) if subdural bleed and diffuse axonal injury combined
- Amount of blood that is significant dependent on age and rapidity of accumulation
  - Infant—a few milliliters
  - Children (1–3 yr)–30 mL
  - Adult–100–150 mL
- May be categorized based on the interval between the hematoma and the traumatic event
  - Acute: within 3 d of trauma
  - Subacute: between 3 d and 3 wk post-trauma
  - Chronic: develops after 3 wk
- Microscopic dating of subdural hematoma
  - 1 wk—lysis of clot
  - 2 wk—growth of fibroblasts from the dural surface into the hematoma
  - 1–3 mos—early development of hyalinized connective tissue

C. Subarachnoid hemorrhage

- May be related to trauma
- Nontraumatic causes most commonly the result of saccular aneurysm and vascular malformation
- May be secondary to contiguous rupture of intraparenchymal hemorrhage
- Traumatic basilar subarachnoid hemorrhage following a blow to the face, jaw, or neck—result of tear of vertebral artery at C1

III. Skull Fractures

A. Classification

- Will be present, by definition, in an open or penetrating head wound
- May be present in up to 80% of fatal closed head injuries
- Fractures should be located accurately (i.e., calvarium, base of skull, facial bones) and defined as to the type
  - Linear
  - Depressed (displaced)
  - Diastatic
  - Open or closed
  - Comminuted—bone fragmented
  - Compound fracture with skull laceration overlying the fracture

B. Linear skull fractures

- AKA bursting fractures
- Make up the majority of skull fractures
- Secondary to the "outbending" of the skull at a point distant from the traumatic impact
- Frequently seen in falls and traffic accidents
- Diastatic fractures—subset of linear fractures occurring in young people, defined as linear fractures that cause separation of or across cranial sutures

C. Depressed skull fractures

- Secondary to low-velocity local traumatic forces, also called bending fractures
- Subdivided into stellate and comminuted
- Depressed skull fracture present if the inner table of the skull is depressed by a distance equal to the thickness of the skull or greater
  - Further subdivided into open or closed

based on the presence or absence of an overlying scalp laceration

- Most common in the frontal or parietal region
- Rule of thumb: If the fracture is below the hat brim, it is more likely to be secondary to a fall; a fracture above the hat brim level is more likely secondary to traumatic force
- Two special types of depressed skull fracture: orbital blow-in and blow-out fractures
  - Occur in elderly people who have sustained a blow to the back or top of the head
  - May represent contrecoup movement of the frontal lobes over the thin bones in the frontal fossa

D. Basilar skull fractures

- Common, difficult to diagnose by x-ray
- Must strip dura from the skull base to visualize, when basilar fracture is suspected at autopsy
- Result of significant force from falls, motor vehicle accidents, or assaults
- Subtypes include hinge, ring, and contracoup fractures
- Battle sign—soft tissue swelling and discoloration in the area of the mastoid, secondary to blood in the mastoid air cells
- Raccoon eyes—represents periorbital ecchymoses, may be seen with basilar skull fractures

E. Hinge fractures

- Special type of fracture
- Occur with crushing injuries, such as compression of the head between the ground and a heavy object (i.e., a car tire)
- May be either longitudinal or transverse
- Transverse hinge fracture extends across the dorsum sellae of the skull

IV. Contusions

A. General characteristics

- Most characteristic lesions of trauma
- Contusions are parenchymal brain injuries
  - Typically wedge shaped and preferentially affect the crown of the gyri
  - Most common sites frontal and temporal poles

○ In many contusions, the pial–glial membrane disrupted; by definition, the contusion then accompanied by a laceration

- A fracture contusion may develop at site of fracture

- Hernation contusion represents bruising of the uncus and/or parahippocampal gyrus as it impacts on the dura of the tentorial notch; produced by sudden, forceful herniation of brain tissue

- Gliding contusion—focal hemorrhage in cortex and underlying white matter at the superior margins of the cerebral hemispheres, usually bilateral but asymmetrical

B. Coup and contrecoup contusions

- Coup lesions—contusions immediately beneath and associated with direct trauma

  ○ Stationary head impacted by object that deforms the skull and impacts enough energy to damage the underlying brain surface

  ○ Skull must be intact (i.e., no fractures)

- Contrecoup lesions—contusions at a distance from and frequently roughly opposite to the point of trauma

  ○ Often represent rotational brain movement and deceleration injury

  ○ Thought to be related to the irregularities of the skull opposite the point of impact

  ○ "Burst lobe"—pulped frontal or temporal pole resulting from massive contrecoup contusion, associated with subdural hemorrhage

V. Other Lesions

A. Penetrating versus perforation wounds

- Penetrating brain wounds—the object enters but does not completely transverse the brain (stab wounds, low-velocity gunshot)

- Perforating brain wounds—wounds in which the object passes through the brain and exits

- Factors to keep in mind related to brain wounds:

  ○ Entrance wound (marginal abrasion, muzzle imprint, soot, stippling)

  ○ Exit wound

  ○ Internal ricochet—lower-velocity bullets

○ Cavitation

○ Secondary missile production—pieces of bone break off

- Gunshot wounds

  ○ Wounding capacity related to velocity of missile

  ○ Tissue damage resulting from track of bullet and temporary cavity that follows the bullet (damage from stretching in adjacent tissue)

  ○ Entrance wound through skull will have a broader inner table bevel; exit will have a broader outer table bevel

B. Blunt head injury

- Static loading—forces are applied to the head gradually (more than 200 ms to develop) (e.g., earthquakes or landslides)

- Dynamic loading—forces are applied < 200 ms

  ○ Impulsive loading—head is set in motion or moving head is stopped without being struck (blows to face and thorax)

  ○ Impact loading—blunt object strikes head, injury often related to both contact and inertia factors

  ○ Strain caused by loading is the cause of tissue injury as a result of compression, tension, or shear

- May be accompanied by skin lesions

  ○ Abrasions—scraping away of skin surface (scratches, brush burns)

  ○ Contusions—bruise (extravasation of blood into soft tissue)

  ○ Ecchymoses—extravasation of blood from one site to another

    ▶ Periorbital (raccoon eyes)—fractures of orbital plates of the anterior cranial fossa

    ▶ Mastoid (battle sign) fracture of petrous bone lacerating the internal carotid artery

  ○ Laceration—splitting or tearing of the tissue

- Crushing head injury—stationary head impacted by massive force that crushes the skull, brain often lacerated by bone fragments and fracture contusions

- Infant brains
  - Smooth skull base and pliable skull
  - Contusion tears—separation of cortex from subcortical white matter
  - Coup and contrecoup contusions seldom seen in children before age 3–4 yr

C. Diffuse axonal injury
- AKA: intermediary coup lesions, Strich lesions
- Shearing injury of nerve fibers
- Associated with traffic accidents (frontal, occipital or vertex impacts) and shaken infants
- Deformation of brain in the anterior–posterior direction
- Damage to corpus callosum, fornix, corona radiata, superior cerebellar peduncles

- Punctate or streak-like hemorrhages
- Axonal injury—retraction balls or spheroids (seen on silver stain), seen as early as 4–12 h after injury
- May get avulsion of the pontomedullary or cervicomedullary junction with severe hyperextension of neck
- May result from angular acceleration

D. Fat emboli
- Fracture of long bones
- Fat globules in circulation
- Often presents with sudden onset tachypnea, dyspnea, and tachycardia 1–3 d after injury
- Petechial white matter hemorrhages
- Need to process tissue fresh to stain with oil-red-O or lipid stain

5 Congenital Malformations, Perinatal Disease, and Phacomatoses

I. Congenital Malformations

A. Disorders of closure

- AKA: dysraphism
- Closure of neural tube (4th wk)
- Craniorachischisis totalis—total failure of closure
  - Brain and cord exposed to amniotic fluid
  - Necrosis and degeneration of brain and cord
- Anencephaly
  - AKA: exencephalia acrania
  - Defective closure of anterior end of neural tube
  - Most aborted prematurely
  - Females > males, high incidence in Ireland and Wales
  - Associated cranial vault and scalp defects
  - Base of skull thickened, flattened; sphenoid wing abnormalities, shallow orbits
  - Brain absent or rudimentary (cystic mass with vessels—area cerebrovasculosa)
  - Eyes well formed (optic vesicles form very early)
  - Cerebellum and brain stem may be present, but usually absent
  - Absence or hypoplasia of pituitary (50%)
  - Amyelia—total absence of cord
- Cranium bifidum with encephalocele
  - Protrusion of brain and meninges through congenital opening of skull
  - Result of failure of overlying mesenchymal tissue to develop
  - Posterior type (midoccipital, occipitocervical) most common in fatal cases
  - Occipital encephalocele is part of Meckel-Gruber syndrome—autosomal recessive condition with sloping forehead, polydactyly, polycystic kidneys, and hepatic fibrosis
- Spina bifida
  - Meningocele—subcutaneous herniation of meninges through defective closure of vertebral arch
  - Meningomyelocele—herniation of both leptomeninges and cord through a vertebral defect
    - Often associated with hydrocephalus, Chiari type II malformation, and other spinal cord anomalies (syringomyelia, hydromyelia, diastematomyelia)
    - Lesions above T12 level more likely associated with other malformations and more common in females
  - Myelocystocele—myelomeningocele with central canal dilatation and thin posterior cord
  - Myeloschisis—cleft cord with interposed vascular tissue with remnants of neural tissue

- Diastematomyelia—cord segments separated by collagen or bone, 50% associated with myeloschisis and myelocystocele, rarely extends above the mid-thoracic levels

- Diplomyelia—duplication of the spinal cord

- Aqueductal malformations

  - Stenosis without gliosis

  - Forking

  - Septum (neuroglial membrane)—obstructing caudal end

  - Gliosis—narrowing or subdivision of aqueduct

  - Acquired destructive process

- Hydromyelia

  - Congenital dilatation of central canal

  - Associated with meningomyelocele and Chiari malformation

  - Rarely symptomatic

- Syringomyelia

  - Slit or tubular cavitation of cord (syrinx = tube)

  - Most commonly cervical or thoracic cord

  - Cavity may be multiple, irregular

  - May be filled with fluid associated with compression and damage to surrounding tissue

  - Histology—variable, cavity resembles tear, may see astrocytosis

  - Associated with intramedullary tumors

- Syringobulbia

  - Cavity in medulla

  - Often associated with cervical syringomyelia

B. Disorders of diverticulation

- Holoprosencephaly

  - AKA: holotelencephaly (failure of anterior telencephalon to divide [i.e. incomplete separation of the cerebral hemispheres across the midline])

  - Associated with trisomy 13 and increased risk in diabetic mother

  - Associated craniofacial malformations

    - Cyclopia

    - Nasal protuberance or proboscis above orbits

    - Agnathia (absence of jaw)

    - Fusion of ears

    - Situs inversus

    - Cleft lip/palate

    - Trigonocephaly

  - Three types

    - Alobar

      ▷ Most severe form

      ▷ Monoventricular small cerebrum remains undivided into lobes

      ▷ Thin membrane forms a portion of ventricle roof

      ▷ Absent olfactory bulbs and tracts

      ▷ Associated facionasal malformations

      ▷ Brain stem and cerebellum generally normal

    - Semilobar

      ▷ Incomplete lobe formation

      ▷ Partial formation of a shallow interhemispheric fissure

      ▷ Absent olfactory bulb tracts

      ▷ Associated facionasal malformation

    - Lobar

      ▷ Lobes and interhemispheric fissures well formed

      ▷ Ocular abnormalities

      ▷ Usually normal karyotype, 13–15 trisomy

- Chiari malformations

  - Type I (adult)

    - Downward herniation of cerebellar tonsils

    - No elongation of medulla and 4th ventricle

    - No associated spina bifida

    - Often asymptomatic, may cause late onset hydrocephalus

    - Arachnoidal adhesions

    - Associated with syringomyelia (50%)

  - Type II (infantile)

- ► Malformation of basocranial bones
  - ▷ Platybasia (flattened)
  - ▷ Occipito-atlantal assimulation (fusion)
  - ▷ Small foramen magnum
  - ▷ Cervical spina bifida
  - ▷ Klippel-Feil abnormality (vertebral fusion)
  - ▷ Craniolacunia—irregular patches of cranial vault thinning or erosion
- ► Cerebellar malformations
- ► Persistence of embryonic cervical flexure
  - ▷ Foreshortening of hindbrain
  - ▷ Elongation and downward displacement of inferior vermis, medulla, and cervical cord
- ► Associated features
  - ▷ Lumbar meningocele or meningomyelocele (95%)
  - ▷ Hydrocephalus (95%)
  - ▷ Microgyria (55%)
  - ▷ Tectal malformation (75%)
  - ▷ Aqueductal atresia (>35%)
- o Type III
  - ► Very rare
  - ► Occipitocervical or high cervical bony defect with herniation of cerebellum through the defect
- o Dandy-Walker syndrome
  - ► Hypoplasia or aplasia of cerebellar vermis
  - ► Cystic dilatation of 4th ventricle
  - ► Enlargement of posterior fossa
  - ► Hydrocephalus symptoms early, prominent occiput
  - ► Variable agenesis of corpus callosum, neuronal heterotopia, spinal dysplasia, renal defects, polydactylism, pachygyria, polymicrogyria, microcephaly, aqueduct stenosis, syringomyelia, meningocele, spina bifida
  - ► Compatible with normal life
- C. Disorders of neuronal migration
  - • Cortical dysplasia

- o Most develop by the 16th wk of gestation
- o Miller-Dieker syndrome—del 17p13.3 (LIS-1 gene, seizures, mental retardation, and agyria)
- o Gross patterns include agyria, pachygyria polymicrogyria, hemimegalencephaly, nodular and laminar heterotopias
- o All marked by an abnormal arrangement of neurons in the cortex
- o Several histologic types
  - ► Laminar architecture abnormalities
  - ► Neuronal disorientation within cortex
  - ► Hypercellular molecular layer
  - ► Balloon cells
  - ► Neuronal dysmorphism
  - ► Pial–arachnoidal glioneuronal heterotopia
  - ► Neuronal cytomegaly
- • Association with tuberous sclerosis, neurofibromatosis type I, epidermal nevus syndrome
- • Association with neoplasia (ganglioglioma, dysembryoplastic neuroepithelial tumor [DNT])
- • Neuronal heterotopia
  - o White matter neurons
  - o Frequently seen in epilepsy patients
  - o Significance uncertain
- D. Disorders of sulcation
  - • Normal development
    - o 5th mo—first fissures form
    - o 3rd trimester—secondary sulci form
    - o 3rd trimester to 6 mo of age—tertiary sulci form
  - • Lissencephaly (agyria) and pachygyria
    - o Agyria—absence of convolution
    - o Pachygyria—few broad gyri
    - o Bilateral or unilateral
    - o Associated with neuronal migration abnormalities between 11th and 13th wk of gestation
    - o Brain small, underweight (microcephalus vera)

- Lateral ventricles larger (colpocephaly)

- Decrease in number of secondary gyri

- Depth of gray matter underlying the smooth part of cortex increased

- Calvaria usually small, misshaped and thick

- Microscopic cortical dysplasia, four-layer cortex

- Often with heterotopias

- Associated with small jaw, severe mental and motor retardation, failure to thrive, seizures

- Walker-Warburg syndrome (HARD + E syndrome)

  ▶ Hydrocephalus, agyria, retinal dysplasia, encephalocele

  ▶ Psychomotor retardation severe, death in infancy

- Cerebro-ocular dysplasia—muscular dystrophy syndrome

  ▶ Similar to Walker-Warburg syndrome plus muscle disease

  ▶ Muscular dystrophy

- Neu-Laxova syndrome

  ▶ Agyria with microcephaly

  ▶ Autosomal recessive

  ▶ May also see intrauterine growth retardation, skin dysplasia, organ hypoplasia, facial anomalies

- Micropolygyria (polymicrogyria)

  - Miniature, incomplete convolution

  - Abnormal cortical architecture (four-layer cortex, absent molecular layer), thin cortical ribbon

  - Associated with cerebellar microgyria

  - Associated with neuronal migration abnormalities between 20th and 24th wk of gestation.

  - Zellweger's syndrome

    ▶ Microgyria and polymicrogyria

    ▶ Peroxisome abnormality

    ▶ Chromosomes 1, 7, and 8

E. Disorders of proliferation

- Megalencephaly

- Excessive weight (1600–2850 g), brain weight 2.5 standard deviations above the mean for age and gender

- Heavy brain with associated anomalies

- Three types

  ▶ Diffuse blastomatous glial overgrowth—associated with malignancy and dysplasia

  ▶ Increased size without glial proliferation

  ▶ Increased size secondary to other disease (tuberous sclerosis, Tay-Sachs, leukodystrophies such as Alexander's disease)

- Megalocephaly—enlargement of head

- Microencephaly

  - < 900 g weight in adults

  - Associated microcephaly (small head)

  - Most the result of perinatal destructive processes

  - Familial type (500–600 g), recessive defect

- Schizencephaly

  - Symmetrical clefts in line of primary fissures and involve whole depth of cerebral wall

  - Two types

    ▶ Clefts intact

    ▶ Internal hydrocephalus, clefts covered by membrane

  - Clefts resulting from localized failure of growth and differentiation in cerebral wall before end of 2nd mo of gestation

F. Disorders of commissuration

- Agenesis of corpus callosum

  - 12–22 wk of gestation

  - Asymptomatic or associated with mental retardation, seizures, speech disturbances

  - Associated with holoprosencephaly, pachygyria, schizencephaly

  - Associated with webbed toes, funnel chest, spina bifida, persistent fontanelles, facial asymmetry, high arched palate, agenesis of cerebellar vermis, ventricular septal defect

- Abnormalities of septum pellucidum
  - Agenesis/hypoplasia
    - Associated with agenesis of corpus callosum, holoprosencephaly, defects of lateral ventricles and optic nerve
  - Cavum septi pellucidi
    - Normal in newborn, separation of the leaflets of the septum pellucidum
    - Asymptomatic

G. Trisomies
  - Down's syndrome (Trisomy 21)
    - Brain more rounded (reduced frontal lobe)
    - Usually decreased brain weight
    - Narrowing of superior temporal gyrus; bilateral in half of cases
    - Brain stem and cerebellum small versus cerebrum
    - Loss of neurons focally (cortical layer 3), poor myelination
    - Alzheimer's disease-like changes in middle-aged patients
    - May see pathology in brain (abscess, embolic disease) related to congenital heart abnormalities that can be seen in Down's syndrome
  - Patau syndrome (Trisomy 13)
    - Holoprosencephaly and arhinencephaly < 2/3 of cases
    - May see cyclopia, microcephaly, and cerebellar dysplasia
  - Edward's syndrome (Trisomy 18)
    - Microcephaly, dysplasia, disorganization of the lateral geniculate nucleus

H. Cerebellar malformations
  - Total agenesis rare, often associated with hypoplastic/dysplastic pontine nuclei and inferior olives; may see with large occipital encephaloceles
  - Aplasia of vermis
    - Seen in Dandy-Walker syndrome
    - Joubert syndrome
      - Episodic hyperpnea, abnormal eye movements, ataxia, mental retardation

  - ▶ Cerebral hemispheres largely unaffected
  - ▶ 4th ventricle dilated
- Pontoneocerebellar hypoplasia
  - Microcephaly
  - Hypoplastic cerebellar hemispheres
  - Dentate nuclei disorganized
  - Death by age 2 yr
- Granular cell aplasia
- Cerebellar heterotopia—ectopic gray matter in cerebellar white matter, more common in hemispheres
- Cerebellar cortical dysplasia—disorganized cerebellar cortical architecture

I. Brain stem malformations
  - Olivary heterotopia
  - Olivary and dentate dysplasia

J. Hippocampal sclerosis (mesial temporal sclerosis)
  - Associated with chronic epilepsy
  - Neuronal cell loss and gliosis in Sommer sector region (CA1), dentate and endplate (CA4) of hippocampus
  - Etiology uncertain

II. Perinatal Pathology
  A. Perinatal lesions of CNS
    - "Birth injuries"—may be misnomer
    - Uncertainty regarding time of insult
    - Types
      - Anoxic/ischemic
      - Trauma
      - Infection
      - Toxic/metabolic
  B. Anoxia/ischemia
    - Prenatal causes include maternal anemia, heart disease, pneumonia, shock, placental abnormality (umbilical cord knots, infarcts, infection), multiple gestations (twins, triplets, etc.)
    - Oversedation (improper anesthesia at delivery)
    - Postnatal causes include aspiration, unrelieved airway obstruction, respiratory distress syndrome, pneumonia

C. Ulegyria
- Related to cortical ischemia
- Shrunken sclerotic gyri
- Loss of tissue at sulci depth
- Watershed areas
- Flanked by gyri with less neuronal loss and irregular patches of myelinated axons

D. Diffuse lobar sclerosis
- Related to cortical ischemia
- Evenly distributed atrophy
- Bilateral, symmetrical
- "Walnut kernel brain"
- Secondary white matter atrophy

E. Basal gray matter necrosis
- Related to ischemia
- Cystic necrosis
- Partial necrosis
  - Irregular neuronal loss and astrocytosis
  - Overgrowth of perivascular myelinated nerve fibers (status marmoratus, état marblé), ferruginization of residual neurons

F. Multilocular cystic encephalomalacia
- Related to ischemia
- Infancy
- Cystic cavities with gliotic white matter remnants

G. Periventricular leukomalacia
- Related to ischemia
- Multifocal, sharply circumscribed foci of necrosis, typically adjacent to lateral ventricle
- Coagulative necrosis starting 3–8 hr after insult, marked by nuclear pyknosis, edema, eosinophilia, swollen axons (spheroids)
- After 12–15 hr, marginal astrocytic proliferation and capillary hyperplasia seen
- Microglial proliferation and macrophages within 1 wk
- Later astrocytosis, mineralized axons, cavitation
- Associated with prematurity (greatest risk 28–32 wk), respiratory distress syndrome, apnea, cardiac arrest
- Petechiae, hemorrhage in white matter
- Perinatal telencephalic leukoencephalopa-

thy–hypertrophic astrocytes, perivascular globules in white matter, Gram-negative endotoxin effect on myelin formation

H. Hydranencephaly
- Related to ischemic change
- Cerebral hemispheres (carotid distribution)—membranous sacs of leptomeninges and gliosis
- Porencephaly—continuation with ventricular system and subarachnoid space
- Spastic quadriplegia, failure to develop

I. Germinal matrix hemorrhage
- Cause: perinatal anoxia
- Prematurity increased risk, <32 wk
- Rupture of thin-walled veins related to congestion
- Intraventricular hemorrhage
- Cavitary lesions in healed cases
- May see choroid plexus hemorrhage (full term)

J. Subarachnoid hemorrhage
- Origin
  - Related to germinal matrix bleed into ventricle
  - De novo related to anoxia
  - Traumatic venous tear
- Progressive hydrocephalus
- May see in cerebellum

K. Perinatal vascular lesions
- Arterial
  - Thrombotic occlusions rare (middle cerebral artery most common site)
  - Embolic—congenital heart disease
- Venous
  - Circulatory failure and leptomeningitis—stasis thrombosis
  - Premature—deep internal venous system
  - Term—superficial cerebral veins and sinuses
- Arteriovenous malformation

L. Subdural hemorrhage
- Trauma related, full term with prolonged labor
- Laceration of falx or tentorium

- Damage to bridging veins, straight sinus, vein of Galen
- Posterior fossa rare, more serious than convexity
- Subdural hygroma—hematoma encased by neomembrane

M. Ponto-subicular necrosis

- Neuronal necrosis in basis pontis ± subiculum
- Pathogenesis may be function of disordered flow through vertebrobasilar circulation

N. Möbius syndrome

- Necrosis of selected cranial nerve nuclei (especially VI and VII)
- Destruction may occur *in utero* or in neonatal period
- Masked facies (facial diplegia) and strabismus
- Skeletal abnormalities and mental retardation

O. Bilirubin encephalopathy

- AKA: kernicterus, nuclear jaundice
- Associated with erythroblastosis fetalis, hemolytic anemias
- Two patterns
    - Symmetrical; pallidum, substantia nigra, Ammon's horn, cranial nerve nuclei (III, VIII, XII), inferior olive, dentate
    - Diffuse, associated with periventricular leukomalacia
- Damage to blood-brain barrier with necrosis
- Discoloration of neurons (lost over time), pyknosis, eosinophilic neuronal degeneration, glial scarring, atrophy
- Increased risk with low albumin, respiratory distress, acidosis

P. Alcohol (fetal alcohol syndrome)

- Dysraphism
- Holoprosencephaly
- Agenesis of corpus callosum
- Porencephaly
- Microcephaly
- Hydrocephalus
- Cerebellar malformations
- Optic nerve hypoplasia
- Retinal ganglion cell loss
- Cortical dysplasia

III. Phacomatoses

A. Neurofibromatosis type I (classical type NF-I, von Recklinghausen's disease)

- Autosomal dominant, 1 : 3000–1 : 5000
- 50% of cases are sporadic
- Variable expressivity and penetrance
- Gene located chromosome 17q11.2
- Gene product: neurofibromin, a GTP-ase activating protein
- Diagnostic criteria for NF-I (need at least two of the following)
    - Six or more café-au-lait macules >5 mm in diameter in children and >15 mm in teenagers and adults (usually present at birth or early childhood, flat and hyperpigmented macules)
    - At least two neurofibromas of any type or one plexiform neurofibroma
    - Axillary or inguinal freckling (intertriginous hyperpigmentation)
    - Optic nerve glioma (12% of NF-I patients, 50% of childhood tumors are in patients with NF-I)
    - Two or more hamartomas of the iris (Lisch nodules) (mostly bilateral, appear by age 2–5 yr by slit-lamp exam)
    - A distinct osseous lesion (sphenoid dysplasia, thinning of long-bone cortex with or without pseudoarthrosis).
    - A first-degree relative (parent, sibling or child) with NF-I
- Other findings may include malignant peripheral nerve sheath tumor, meningioangiomatosis, pheochromocytoma, cranial and renal artery stenosis, skull defects, rhabdomyosarcoma, Wilm's tumor and nonlymphocytic leukemia, glioma, dural ectasia, macrocephaly, cortical dysplasia/hamartomas, scoliosis/kyphosis

B. Neurofibromatosis type II (central type, NF-II)

- Autosomal dominant
- 1 : 50,000
- Mutation rare
- Gene located chromosome 22q
- Gene product: merlin (a cytoskeletal protein

and tumor suppressor)—moesin–ezrin–radixin-like protein

- Diagnostic criteria (need one of following)
  - Bilateral cranial nerve VIII masses seen with appropriate imaging (schwannoma)
  - A first-degree relative with NF-II and either a unilateral cranial nerve VIII mass or two of the following:
    - ▶ Neurofibroma
    - ▶ Meningioma
    - ▶ Glioma
    - ▶ Schwannoma
    - ▶ Juvenile posterior subcapsular lenticular opacity

C. Tuberous sclerosis
- "Tuber"-potato-like growth, lesions often calcify with age—"sclerotic"
- Autosomal dominant with incomplete penetrance; 6 : 100,000 incidence
- Frequently sporadic (50–80%)
- Forme-fruste cases common
- Decreased life expectancy
- Chromosome 9q34 (TSC1 gene) and 16 p13.3 (TSC2 gene)
- Classic triad: adenoma sebaceum, seizures, mental retardation
- Tuberous sclerosis findings in central nervous system
  - Subependymal giant-cell astrocytoma, usually near foramen of Monro
  - Astrocytic hamartomas—small nodules, "candle guttering," lateral ventricles
  - "Tubers"—firm, ill-defined, widened gyri, disorganized cortical architecture, can calcify, sheaf-like bundles of neuroglial fibers in superficial part of tuber
  - "Idiopathic" ventricular dilatation
  - Cortical dysplasia
  - Seizures in 90% of patients
  - Mental retardation in a minority of patients
- Tuberous sclerosis findings in other organ systems
  - Adenoma sebaceum (angiofibroma)—60–90% of patients over 4 yr of age
  - Shagreen patches—lumbar and intertriginous areas of leathery macular patches, 20% of patients
  - Ash-leaf patches—hypopigmented patches
  - Periungual fibromas—5–50% of patients
  - Angiomyolipoma
  - Polycystic kidneys in children
  - Cardiac rhabdomyomas
  - Lymphangioleiomyomatosis
  - Retinal hamartoma

D. Sturge-Weber disease
- AKA: encephalotrigeminal angiomatosis
- Absence of familial predisposition
- Facial port wine stain (nevus flammeus)—especially trigeminal region
- Seizures, retardation
- Leptomeningeal venous angioma
- Cortical calcification (tram-line type of calcification radiologically) and atrophy
- Hemihypertrophy of skull—reaction to brain atrophy, elevation of sphenoid wing and petrous ridges, enlarged paranasal sinuses
- Congenital buphthalmus and glaucoma
- Hemiatrophy of body—contralateral to facial nevus, result of hemiparesis

E. von Hippel-Lindau disease
- 1/31,000–1/53,000 incidence
- 20% of cases with familial incidence, males > females
- Autosomal dominant with incomplete penetrance, chromosome 3p
- Cerebellar hemangioblastoma (Lindau's tumor) and retinal hemangioblastoma (von Hippel's disease)
- Renal cell carcinoma and renal cysts
- Hepatic adenomas and cysts
- Pancreatic adenoma
- Epididymal cystadenoma
- Pheochromocytoma
- Polycythemia associated with hemangioblastoma
- Paragangliomas
- Aggressive papillary tumor of middle ear

F. Ataxia—telangiectasia

- 1/40,000 incidence
- Autosomal recessive
- Chromosome 11q22–23
- Progressive cerebellar ataxia (usually presents in infancy), conjunctival and facial telangiectasias, immunoglobulin abnormalities [especially IgA], hypersensitivity to radiation, predisposition to lymphoma, thymus absent or rudimentary, hypoplastic gonads)
- Abnormality of DNA processing and repair
- Cerebellar cortical atrophy as a result of defective maturation of Purkinje cells and granular neurons, posterior column degeneration, nuclear pleomorphism and cytoplasmic enlargement in Schwann cells and ganglionic satellite cells

G. Neurocutaneous melanosis (Touraine syndrome)

- Autosomal dominant
- Melanocytic proliferation of leptomeninges, skin, and eye
- Some cases sporadic
- Rarely associated with neurofibromatosis

H. Cowden syndrome

- Dysplastic gangliocytoma of cerebellum (Lhermitte-Duclos)
- Also develops trichilemmomas, hamartomas, benign tumors of the skin and other organs, thyroid carcinoma

I. Retinoblastoma syndrome

- Prone to developing osteosarcomas, pineoblastomas, malignant gliomas
- Chromosome 13q14, RB1 gene
- Gene product causes cell cycle arrest
- Both normal alleles of Rb locus must be inactivated ("two hits") for development of tumor. In familial cases, the child is born with one normal and one defective copy of the Rb gene. The intact gene copy is lost through a somatic mutation.

J. Li-Fraumeni syndrome

- Malignant gliomas of CNS
- Also predisposed to breast carcinoma, soft tissue sarcoma, osteosarcoma, leukemia, lymphoma, and adrenocortical carcinoma
- *p53* gene on chromosome 17p13

K. Turcot syndrome

- Medulloblastoma and malignant glioma
- Also develop polyposis coli
- Chromosome 5q21, APC gene

L. Gorlen syndrome

- Medulloblastoma
- AKA: basal cell nevus syndrome (basal cell carcinoma), keratocysts of the jaw, ovarian fibromas
- Chromosome 9q31

6 Demyelinating and Dysmyelinating Diseases

I. Demyelinating Disease

  A. Definition

- AKA: myelinoclastic disease
- Disease of central and peripheral nervous system characterized by a selective loss of myelin with relative sparing of axons
- To be distinguished from dysmyelinating disease (i.e., leukodystrophies), which are characterized by loss of myelin with an accumulation of abnormal myelin breakdown products and axonal involvement

  B. Myelin sheath

- Formed by modification of oligodendroglial cell membrane
- 75% lipid, 25% protein
- Myelin basic protein
- Membrane lipids—cholesterol (43%), phospholipids (40%), sphingolipids (17%)

  C. Causes/mechanisms of demyelination

- Oligodendroglial cell affected
  - Viral
  - Chemical
- Myelin affected
  - Immune
  - Viral
  - Chemical
  - Physical

  D. Multiple sclerosis

- Relapses and remissions
- Two-thirds with continuous deterioration
- Subgroups are either rapidly fatal or "benign"
- Genetic predisposition
  - 15–20× risk in immediate relatives
  - 533× risk for identical twins
  - 259× risk for fraternal twins
  - Northern European HLA-DR15
  - Association with M3 antitrypsin allele
  - Geographical distribution
  - High-frequency zones: northern Europe and United States, Southern Canada, New Zealand, southeast Australia; infrequent in Orientals
  - Multiple sclerosis factor operates during adolescence
- Classic clinical presentation
  - Peak age 20–40 yr, females > males
  - Clinical course highly variable
  - Paresthesias, limb weakness, ataxia, bladder dysfunction, nystagmus, optic neuritis, rarely clinically silent
  - Recovery from acute relapse may be the result of loss of edema, decreased astrocytic swelling, disappearance of locally produced substances that interfere with nerve conduction
  - CSF fluid with elevated protein; increased γ-globulin and oligoclonal bands

- Gross pathology

  - May see atrophy

  - Plaques firm, deep white matter, often multiple

    - Diffuse distribution especially periventricular region, optic nerve, spinal cord

    - Cervical cord most common spinal site

- Lesions often of different histologic age

- Acute lesion—myelin fragmentation, relative axonal preservation, microglial proliferation

- Subacute plaque—Loss of myelin and oligodendrocytes, macrophages, free neutral fat, astrocytosis, perivascular lymphocyte inflammation (T-cells)

- Remote/inactive lesion—loss of myelin, some axons and astrocytic processes remain, meningeal inflammation, iron deposits at edge, adjacent white matter abnormal

- Shadow plaques—border between normal and affected white matter where there are abnormally thin myelin sheaths, may represent either partial/incomplete myelin loss or remyelination by surviving oligodendrocytes

- May occasionally see plaques in the cerebral cortex

- Marburg type

  - Acute, fulminant multiple sclerosis

  - Death, often between 1 and 6 mo after onset of symptoms

  - Most plaques histologically acute/subacute (hypercellular)

- Baló type

  - "Concentric sclerosis"

  - Acute onset, typically 2nd and 3rd decades

  - Most patients die in less than 2 yr from presentation

  - Concentric demyelination

- Schilder type

  - Acute/subacute form with one or more large plaques involving cerebral hemisphere and measuring >2 × 3 cm

  - Seen predominantly in childhood

- Dévic type

  - "Neuromyelitis optica"

  - Blindness with paraplegia (demyelination of optic nerve and spinal cord)

  - Most with acute onset, 50% die within months of clinical onset

E. Tumor-like demyelinating lesion

- Most present with a solitary lesion, radiographically suggesting tumor

- Subset of patients are older (i.e., >55 yr)

- Most improve with steroid therapy, most do not develop additional lesions

- Pathology marked by demyelination (white matter macrophages, reactive astrocytosis, perivascular chronic inflammation)

F. Acute disseminated encephalomyelitis

- Postvaccination, postinfectious (measles, mumps, chicken pox, rubella, whooping cough, herpes simplex)

- Sudden onset 5–14 d after viral infection or immunization

- Generally good prognosis, death 10%

- Immunological mechanism (resembles experimental allergic encephalitis).

- Pathology marked by perivascular demyelination, perivascular inflammation (acute and chronic), microglial proliferation

- In acute phase, considerable edema (with herniation) and vascular congestion possible

G. Acute hemorrhagic leukoencephalitis

- AKA: Weston-Hurst disease

- Less than age 30 yr, males > females

- Incidence highest in spring and fall

- Abrupt onset, pyrexia, neck stiffness, hemiplegia, seizure, coma, death in a few days

- Preceded by upper respiratory infection in about 50% of cases

- Increased CSF protein, neutrophils

- Etiology: ? immune complex mediated, perivascular immunoglobulin and complement

- Pathology marked by swollen, soft brain, symmetrical white matter hemorrhages, necrosis of vessel wall, perivascular edema, neutrophils, perivascular demyelination, ball and ring hemorrhages (thrombosed capillary in center)

H. Central pontine myelinolysis

- Pons (central part of upper and middle pons), other sites may be affected

- Loss of myelin, preservation of neurons
- Oligodendrocytes lost
- Reactive astrocytosis
- Associated with abnormalities of sodium (rapid increase from hyponatremic state)

I. Marchiafava-Bignami disease
- Corpus callosum and genu demyelination, may see lesions elsewhere
- "Drinkers of crude red wine," associated with alcohol use
- Degeneration of anterior commissure and middle cerebellar peduncles
- Total loss of oligodendrocytes, macrophage and astrocyte response, vessels in involved regions may proliferate and show hyalinized walls
- Pathogenesis not known, toxic?

J. Toxic
- Chronic cyanide
- Chronic methyl alcohol
- Amphotericin B
- Many others

II. Dysmyelinating Diseases
A. Metachromatic leukodystrophy
- Autosomal recessive
- Arylsulfatase A deficiency, chromosome 22q
- Sulfatide accumulation
- Most common form late—infantile
- Diagnosis: amniotic fluid fibroblast assay, leukocytes, urine assay
- Electromyography (EMG) of peripheral nerve abnormal—loss of myelinated axons and thin myelin sheaths
- Onset age 1–2 yr with flaccid weakness, psychomotor retardation, quadriplegia, blindness
- Death in 2 yr
- Adult type presents with psychosis and dementia, may die of venous thrombosis
- Chalky discoloration of white matter, macrophages containing cerebroside sulfate
- Preservation of arcuate fibers
- Severe axonal damage and loss
- Metachromatic granular bodies in macrophages, neurons, Schwann cells
- Metachromasia—when sulfatide binds to certain dyes there is a shift in the absorbance spectrum of the dye
- Electron microscopy
  - Cytoplasmic bodies in oligodendrocytes, astrocytes, Schwann cells, 3 types
    - Concentrically lamellar structures (tuffstone inclusions)
    - Herringbone pattern or hexagonal arrangement
    - Laminated structures or zebra-like bodies
    - Also seen in skin, kidney, liver, gallbladder, and urine

B. Globoid cell leukodystrophy
- AKA: Krabbe's disease
- Autosomal recessive
- Deficiency of galactocerebroside-B galactosidase
- Diagnose with enzyme assay using serum, white blood cells, cultured fibroblasts
- Onset 3–5 mo
- Seizures, feeding problems, hyperirritability, psychomotor retardation, cortical blindness
- Death by age 2 yr
- Cerebral atrophy
- Gray discoloration of centrum ovale and corona radiata
- Spares arcuate fibers
- "Globoid" cell proliferation along vessels, macrophage origin
- Cells PAS positive, weakly sudan positive
- Pyramidal tracts most severely affected
- Reactive astrocytosis
- Loss of large myelinated axons with segmental demyelination
- Electron microscopy: inclusions—straight or curved tubular profiles with longitudinal striations within globoid cells

C. Adrenoleukodystrophy
- Adrenomyeloneuropathy (spastic paraparesis, distal symmetrical polyneuropathy)
- Neonatal
- Symptomatic heterozygote
- Most X-linked (Xq28)
- Classical form with onset in 1st decade

- Visual symptoms early, motor signs later
- Steady deterioration with death in 5 yr
- One-third with adrenocortical failure
- Cutaneous pigmentation
- Some juvenile forms with long survival
- Adults may present with psychiatric symptoms
- Defect in long-chain fatty acid metabolism (carbon chain length >22)
- Firm, gray colored white matter; occipital, parietal, temporal lobes; atrophy symmetric
- Relative sparing of subcortical arcuate fibers, band of Gennari, frontal lobe, brain stem, and spinal cord
- Microscopically three zones
  - Destruction of myelin, axonal sparing, occasional PAS-positive sudanophilic macrophages
  - Myelinated and demyelinated axons, inflammation, and macrophages
  - Dense gliosis, loss of oligodendrocytes, myelin, and axons
- Degeneration of geniculate bodies, hippocampal dentate nucleus
- Electron microscopy: curvilinear inclusions (macrophages)
- Adrenals may show
  - Cortical atrophy, medulla spared
  - Relative sparing of zona glomerulosa
  - Ballooned epithelial cells, lymphs
  - Inclusions—seen in testis (Leydig cells), Schwann cells, nodes, liver, spleen

D. Alexander's disease
- Presents in infancy or childhood
- Progressive dementia, paralysis, epilepsy
- Megalencephalic
- Sporadic
- White cortical ribbon, discolored, loosened white matter
- Diffuse demyelination
- Arcuate fibers not spared
- Rosenthal fibers

E. Canavan's disease
- AKA: van Bogart and Bertrand spongy degeneration
- Deficiency in aspartoacylase
- Subcortical arcuate fibers involved
- Spongy change (spongy degeneration)
- European Jews, autosomal recessive
- Most die in infancy, onset first 6 mo
- Severe mental retardation, head enlargement, hypotonia followed by spastic paralysis
- Demyelination, Alzheimer II astrocytes
- Occipital lobe more involved

F. Pelizaeus-Merzbacher disease
- X-linked—most cases (Xq 21)
- Defect in gene for phospholipid protein
- Classic (type I)
- Onset infantile
- Dementia
- Death within 5 yr
- Atrophic brain
- Brain stem and cerebellum severely affected
- Tigroid demyelination—irregular islands of myelin (perivascular) preserved (some degenerating fibers)
- Astrocytosis

G. Cockayne's disease
- Onset late infancy, autosomal recessive
- Sunken orbits, dwarfism, deafness, mental deficiency, prominent straight nose
- Completely shrunken white matter
- Calcification
- Small brain, atrophic optic nerves, fibrosed meninges

7 Metabolic and Toxic Diseases

I. Metabolic Disorders

   A. Lysosomal disorders

   - Lysosomal enzyme deficiency resulting in accumulation of material in secondary lysosomes.

   - Includes glycogenosis—type II, sphingolipidoses, mucopolysaccharidoses, mucolipidoses, gangliosidoses

   - Others

   B. Tay-Sachs disease

   - GM2 gangliosidosis

   - Autosomal recessive

   - Ashkenazi Jewish population

   - Hexosaminidase A deficiency (lack of synthesis of α-subunit of enzyme)—type B

   - Hexosaminidase A and B deficiency (Sandhoff)—type O, infantile onset

   - Activator protein deficiency, hexosaminidase levels generally normal—Type AB, infantile onset

   - Accumulation of GM2 ganglioside

   - Normal at birth, psychomotor retardation starts after 5–6 mo

   - Later hypotonia and spasticity develop, seizures

   - Brain weight normal or decreased/increased

   - Balloon neurons with cytoplasmic vacuoles

   - Visceral organs generally do not show much evidence of ganglionic accumulation

   - Electron microscopy: whorled membranes or zebra bodies

   - Cherry red spot in macula, blindness

   - Death age 2–3 yr

   - Late infantile form (onset after 18 mo) and rare adult forms exist

   C. GM1 gangliosidosis

   - Infantile form (type I)—failure to thrive, hepatosplenomegaly, facial dysmorphisms, cardiomyopathy, psychomotor retardation, seizures, cherry red spots

   - Late infantile/juvenile (type II)—progressive mental retardation and motor retardation, seizures, death age 3–10 yr, organs normal size

   - Rare adult form (type III)

   - Defect in β-galactosidase (chromosome 3)

   - Brains generally appear grossly normal or atrophic

   - Balloon neuronal cytoplasm with foamy quality and white matter gliosis

   D. Niemann-Pick disease

   - Autosomal recessive, chromosome 11p

   - Mutations common in Ashkenazi Jewish population

   - Sphingomyelinase deficiency (a subset of patients do not have a sphingomyelinase deficiency)

   - Accumulation of sphingomyelin and cholesterol

   - Five phenotypes (A–E)

     ○ Type A—75–80% of cases (severe infantile neurovisceral form)

     ○ Type B—visceral disease only, normal CNS function

   - Electron microscopy: membranous cytoplasmic bodies, zebra bodies

- Brain weight decreased, balloon neurons and glial cells
- Multiorgan involvement with type A, including hepatosplenomegaly, cherry red spots of macula, lung infiltrates
- May see ballooned ganglion cells in the gastrointestinal tract (Auerbach and Meissner plexuses)
- Nieman-Pick cell–foamy phagocyte storage cell seen in extra-CNS organs (sea blue histiocytes)
- Death age 1–2 yr

E. Gaucher's disease
  - Autosomal recessive
  - Glucocerebrosidase deficiency, chromosome 1q
  - Accumulation of glucocerebroside in reticuloendothelial cells and neurons
  - Three clinical types (I: adult, noncerebral; II: infantile, acute cerebral pattern; III: intermediate)
  - Brain gross appearance generally normal
  - Hepatosplenomegaly and lymphadenopathy
  - Gaucher cells (RE cells) rarely vacuolated, fibrillary cytoplasm, "crumpled tissue paper," cells often perivascular in distribution
  - Electron microscopy: distended, elongated lysosomes with stacks of lipid bilayers
  - Neurons shriveled and destroyed, especially cortical layers III and V, Purkinje cells, dentate nucleus

F. Ceroid-lipofuscinoses (Batten's disease)
  - Most autosomal recessive
  - Five main clinical types
    - Infantile type—psychomotor regression starting at about 8 mo, visual loss, hypotonia, ataxia, microcephaly, death age 3–10 yr, chromosome 1p
    - Late infantile type—seizures start between 18 mo and 4 yr, death between 4 and 10 yr
    - Juvenile type—retinopathy presentation between ages 4 and 9 yr, seizures, gait disturbance, hallucinations, death late teens; chromosome 16p
    - Adult type (Kuf's disease)—onset around age 30 yr with myoclonic epilepsy, dementia, ataxia
    - Finnish type—late infantile onset (4–7 yr); chromosome 13q
  - Accumulation of autofluorescent lipopigments in neurons
  - Brain usually atrophic, skull thickened
  - Neuronal loss, gliosis, loss of myelin including subcortical fibers
  - Electron microscopy: granular, curvilinear, fingerprint patterns
  - Biopsy: skin, rectum, or brain to diagnose; can evaluate lymphocytes in some cases

G. Mucopolysaccharidoses
  - Classification
    - Type I Hurler-Scheie; α-L-iduronidase deficiency; chromosome 4p
    - Type II Hunter; iduronate sulfatase deficiency; chromosome Xq
    - Type III Sanfilippo; heparan N-sulfatase, α-N-acetylglucosamindase, acetyl CoA : α-glucosaminide acetyl transferase deficiency; subset with chromosome 12q abnormalities
    - Type IV Morquio; β-galactosidase deficiency; chromosome 16q in subset
    - Type VI Maroteaux-Lamy; N-acetylgalactosaminase-4-sulfatase deficiency; chromosome 5q
    - Type VII Sly; β-glucuronidase deficiency; chromosome 7q
  - Accumulation of dermatan sulfate or heparan sulfates
  - Storage of mucopolysaccharides in lysosomes in multiple organ systems
  - Brains usually grossly normal
  - Perivascular collections of foamy cells, perivascular pitting in white matter
  - Electron microscopy: zebra bodies, membrane-bound lamellar stacks

H. Sialidosis
  - Neuraminidase deficiency; chromosome 10p
  - Cherry red spot of the macula, myoclonus, coarse facial features, skeletal dysplasia, deafness, mental retardation
  - Variable degrees of ballooned neurons, vacu-

olation of neuronal cytoplasm, and lipo-fuscin accumulation

- May see extra-CNS pathology—GI tract, kidney, liver

- A group of disorders (galactosialidoses) marked by a combined neuraminidase/β-galactosidase deficiency

I. Mucolipidoses

- Defect in *N*-acetylglucosamine-1-phospho-transferase; chromosome 4q

- Skull/skeletal deformities, short stature, psychomotor retardation, joint contractures, hepatosplenomegaly (type IV)

- Vacuolated lymphocytes in peripheral blood

- Brain usually normal grossly; may see some neuronal loss and gliosis in type IV

J. Mannosidoses

- Defects in lysosomal α- or β-mannosidase

- Defect in α-mannosidase in autosomal recessive condition, chromosome 19

- Psychomotor retardation, coarse facies, gingival hyperplasia, deafness, hepatosplenomegaly, corneal opacities

- Vacuolation of nerve cells in brain, PAS positive

K. Fucosidosis

- Defect in α-fucosidase; chromosome 1

- Brain may be large or small

- Neuronal ballooning and some neuronal loss/gliosis

- May see many Rosenthal fibers

L. Fabry's disease

- Defect in α-galactosidase A; chromosome Xq

- Skin lesions—telangiectasias (angiokeratoma corporis diffusum)

- Renal insufficiency

- Retinal abnormalities, autonomic dysfunction, hypertrophic cardiomyopathy

- PAS-positive deposits in certain neurons (amygdala, hypothalamus, brain stem)

- Vascular changes in endothelial cells in the brain, infarcts relatively common

- Electron microscopy: lipid lamellae inclusions

M. Cystinosis

- Associated with renal disease, Fanconi's syndrome, photophobia, hypothyroidism

- Widespread deposition of cystine including brain (especially choroid plexus)

- Crystals are soluble, should process tissue fresh/frozen or in alcohol to see crystals on sectioning

N. Lafora body disease

- Abnormality of carbohydrate metabolism resulting in an accumulation of polyglucosan (glucose polymers)

- Autosomal recessive; chromosome 6q

- Seizures with myoclonus

- Microscopically, cytoplasmic neuronal inclusion (Lafora body) with basophilic core and concentric target-like appearance and pale outer zone (PAS positive)

O. Mitochondrial encephalomyopathies

- Leigh's disease

  ○ AKA: subacute necrotizing encephalomyelopathy

  ○ Autosomal recessive disorder

  ○ Lactic acidemia, arrest of psychomotor development, feeding problems, seizures, extraocular palsies, weakness

  ○ Associated with a point mutation at position 8993 of mitochondrial DNA

  ○ Most die within 1–2 yr

  ○ Result of biochemical defects in mitochondrial pathway

  ○ Multifocal, asymmetric destruction of brain tissue

  ○ Vessel proliferation in periventricular gray matter of midbrain, tegmentum of pons, thalamus, and hypothalamus

- MERRF

  ○ Myoclonic epilepsy with ragged red fibers

  ○ Maternally transmitted mitochondrial defect (DNA mutation)

- MELAS

  ○ Mitochondrial encephalopathy, lactic acidosis, and stroke-like episodes

  ○ Mitochondrial abnormalities in cerebral vessels and basal ganglia calcification

P. Phenylketonuria

- Impaired cognitive development
- Can identify patients with neonatal urine screening
- Microcephaly if untreated
- White matter spongiosis and gliosis

Q. Maple syrup urine disease

- Vomiting, lethargy, convulsions, urine smells like maple syrup
- Caused by a variety of defects in α-ketoacid dehydrogenase
- In untreated cases, spongiosis and gliosis of white matter develop

R. Menke's disease

- X-linked recessive disease of copper metabolism
- Mental retardation, hypotonia, hypothermia, visual disturbance, seizures, failure to thrive
- Atrophic brain (especially cerebellum), cerebral arteries thin walled and tortuous (because of altered elastic fibers)
- Neuronal loss and gliosis, hypomyelination, abnormal Purkinje cell dendritic arborization

S. Thiamine deficiency

- Beriberi—associated with a symmetrical peripheral neuropathy (axonal degeneration)
- Wernicke encephalopathy—abrupt onset of psychotic symptoms, if untreated may develop into Korsakoff syndrome marked by memory disturbances and confabulation
- May be caused by any disorder that results in thiamine deficiency (e.g., alcoholism, gastric abnormalites)
- Wernicke encephalopathy marked pathologically by hemorrhage and necrosis of mamillary bodies, periventricular regions, hypothalamic nuclei and thalamus; eventually see gliosis with hemosiderin deposition and macrophages

T. Vitamin B$_{12}$ deficiency

- Subacute combined degeneration of the spinal cord
- Ataxia, numbness and tingling of extremities, spastic weakness/paraplegia of extremities

- Swelling of myelin with vacuolations of thoracic cord with degeneration of posterior columns and descending pyramidal tracts

U. Hepatic encephalopathy

- Alzheimer II astrocytes in cortex and basal ganglia
- Alzheimer II astrocytes—enlarged, pale central chromatin, prominent nuclear membrane and nucleus
- In Wilson's disease (autosomal recessive condition related to copper accumulation), neuronal degeneration in the striatum with Alzheimer II astrocytes

II. Toxic disorders

A. Carbon monoxide

- Selective injury of neurons of layers III and V of cortex, Sommer sector and Purkinje cells
- Bilateral globus pallidus necrosis

B. Methanol

- Edema and petechial hemorrhages
- Degeneration of retinal ganglion cells causing blindness
- Bilateral putamenal necrosis and focal white matter necrosis

C. Ethanol

- Anterior vermal atrophy associated with ataxia and nystagmus
- At risk for developing expressive Wernicke encephalopathy, coagulopathies related to liver disease, head trauma, fetal alcohol syndrome, myelopathy, peripheral neuropathy, central pontine myelinolysis, Marchiafava-Bignami disease

D. Metallic intoxications

- Aluminum—abnormal cytoskeletal derangements, neurofibrillary tangles (structurally different than those of Alzheimer's disease)
- Arsenic—used in weed killers (pesticides), peripheral neuropathy with segmental demyelination, microvascular hemorrhagic encephalopathy in pons and midbrain
- Lead—cerebral edema and vascular congestion, petechial white matter hemorrhages
- Manganese—basal ganglia degeneration (especially medial globus pallidus and substantia nigra)

8 Degenerative Disease

I. Brain Changes in "Normal" Aging
- Loss of mass (10–20%) with neuronal loss
- Ventricular dilatation
- Thickened leptomeninges
- Vascular changes
- Neurofibrillary tangles, neuritic plaques, Lewy bodies, granulovacuolar degeneration, Hirano bodies in small numbers
- Corpora amylacea
- Lipofuscin accumulation
- Increase in astrocyte number and size
- Decrease in neurotransmitters

II. Normal Pressure Hydrocephalus
- Normal CSF pressure
- Elderly
- Triad: dementia, gait disturbance, urinary incontinence
- Ventricular dilatation, no cortical atrophy
- ? impaired CSF absorption
- At autopsy, ventricular size usually decreased (terminal edema, formalin)

III. Alzheimer's Disease
A. General information
- Familial/hereditary cases (5–10%)—begin early, progress rapidly
- Atrophy (temporal, frontal) variable finding
- Impaired higher intellectual function, affect disturbances
- Death usually from infection, inanition, dehydration
- Identical pathologic changes in trisomy 21 patients

B. Proposed causative mechanisms
- Genetic—chromosome 4 (presenilin-1), 21 (amyloid), 19 (apolipoprotein E), 1 (presenilin-2)
- Vascular (amyloidosis)
- Toxic (aluminum)
- Traumatic (head trauma—risk factor)
- Inflammatory (acute-phase reactants)
- Metabolic (mitochondrial abnormality)
- Infection (atypical agent)
- Degenerative (age as risk factor)

C. Gross pathology
- Normal size or atrophic brain
- Atrophy fronto-temporal predisposition (narrowing of gyri and widening of sulci)
- Ventricular dilatation

D. Neuronal loss
- Acetylcholine deficiency
- Nucleus basalis of Meynert—neurons lost, tangles
- Locus ceruleus, nucleus raphe dorsalis, pontine tegmentum, hippocampus and amygdaloid nucleus with variable neuronal loss

E. Neurofibrillary tangles
- Non-membrane-bound masses of filaments
- Silver positive
- Neuronal cytoplasm
- Phosphorylated tau protein (i.e., A68 [tau is a microtubule protein that promotes tubule stability and assembly])

- 10–20-nm filaments in paired helix configuration, crossover every 80 nm
- Tangles may be seen in a whole variety of other pathologies, including normal aging, subacute sclerosing panencephalitis, Niemann Pick disease, Down's syndrome, myotonic dystrophy, dementia pugilistica, progressive supranuclear palsy, Kuf's disease, and Cockayne's syndrome

F. Neuritic plaques

- Spherical structures, 5–200 μm in diameter
- Swollen neurites (dystrophic), contain degenerating clusters of mitochondria, lysosomes, and filaments
- Difficult to see with routine hematoxylin and eosin staining
- The neurites highlighted by silver staining
- β-amyloid core (Congo red, thioflavin S, crystal violet positive), β-amyloid encoded on chromosome 21
- Microglial cells and astrocytosis with amyloid nearby
- Three types
  - Classic/typical
  - Premature—small
  - Burnt out—stellate amyloid with few neurites

G. Granulovacuolar degeneration

- Basophilic granules with halo (3–5 μm)
- Pyramidal neurons of hippocampus
- May represent degenerating autophagocytic process involving cytoskeletal proteins

H. Hirano bodies

- Rod-like or oval eosinophilic cytoplasmic inclusions (10–30 μm in length) within neurons
- May represent abnormal microfilament configurations, by electron microscopy they consist of parallel filaments and sheet-like material

I. Amyloid angiopathy

- Presenilin mutations can cause increased β-amyloid production
- β-Amyloid deposits in cerebral vessel wall (especially in small arteries/arterioles in the leptomeninges and cortex)

- Amorphous/acellular eosinophilic appearance by light microscopy
- β-Amyloid encoded on chromosome 21

J. There are several published pathologic criteria for the diagnosis of Alzheimer's disease

- Khachaturian criteria based on age-related minimum number of senile plaques of neocortex per 1 mm^2 at ×200 magnification
- CERAD (Consortium to Establish a Registry for Alzheimer's Disease) criteria—semiquantitative assessment of plaque frequency in three neocortical regions (superior temporal gyrus, prefrontal cortex, inferior parietal lobule) correlated with age and clinical history of dementia
- Braak and Braak staging—expansion of the CERAD to also evaluate entorhinal cortex and hippocampus, also looks at neurofibrillary tangles

K. Mixed dementia

- One may encounter Alzheimer's disease changes along with other dementia causing pathologies (e.g., diffuse Lewy body disease, Parkinson's disease, infarcts)
- Anywhere between 7% and 25% of Alzheimer's disease patients will have evidence of cerebrovascular disease
- Multi-infarct dementia: >100 mL of infarct, clinically need to be able to temporally relate onset of dementia with stroke

IV. Other Degenerative Disorders

A. Pick's disease

- AKA: lobar atrophy
- Peak age of onset 45–65 yr, uncommon >75 yr
- Less than 2% of dementia cases
- Subset of patients (minority) have autosomal dominant inheritance pattern
- Frontal and temporal lobes preferentially atrophic
- May see atrophy in basal gray nuclei, substantia nigra, outer three layers of cortex
- Neuronal loss, astrocytosis, spongiosis
- "Knife-blade atrophy" or "walnut brain"
- Posterior two-thirds of superior temporal gyrus—spared
- Characteristic pathology marked by balloon cell neurons (Pick cells, globose cells) and

circumscribed argentophilic cytoplasmic inclusions called Pick bodies (silver positive) within neurons consisting of collections of neurofilaments and microtubules. Both Pick cells and Pick bodies stain with antibodies to ubiquitin and tau

B. Huntington's chorea

- Autosomal dominant, gene on short arm of chromosome 4p16.3 (codes for huntingtin); paternal transmission—symptomatic earlier
- Trinucleotide (CAG) repeat disorder
- Choreiform movement, dementia
- Death in 15 yr
- Dopamine activity > acetylcholine activity
- Decrease in choline acetyl-transferase, glutamic acid decarboxylase, and γ-aminobutyric acid
- Pathology
  - ○ Atrophy with loss of small ganglion cells in caudate (tail > body), putamen (anterior > posterior), larger neurons spared
  - ○ Astrocytosis
  - ○ Dilated frontal horns of lateral ventricles, frontal lobe atrophy
  - ○ Nucleus basalis of Meynert spared
  - ○ Vonsattel grading schema
    - ▶ Grade 0—grossly normal, 30–40% neuronal loss in striatum without gliosis
    - ▶ Grade 1—grossly normal, 50% neuronal loss in striatum, gliosis in medial caudate and dorsal putamen
    - ▶ Grade 2—neuronal loss evident in caudate and dorsal putamen with gliosis, gross atrophy of caudate head and putamen
    - ▶ Grade 3—gross atrophy of caudate and putamen and mild atrophy of globus pallidus, neuronal loss as in grade 2, mild astrocytosis of globus pallidus
    - ▶ Grade 4—severe gross atrophy of caudate, putamen, and globus pallidus, microscopic findings worse than grade 3, astrocytosis of nucleus accumbens

C. Parkinson's disease

- AKA: paralysis agitans
- Loss of dopaminergic neurons
- Clinical: pill rolling tremor, rigidity, bradyki-

nesia, disturbance of posture and equilibrium, autonomic dysfunction, dementia (30%); juvenile cases frequently present with dystonia

- Age 45–65 yr
- MPTP-A (contaminant in the illicit synthesis of meperidine analogs); dopamine antagonists cause similar clinical picture
- Most cases idiopathic, some cases with autosomal dominant transmission (linked with α-synuclein gene)
- Mitochondrial dysfunction and free-radical injury may play a role in pathogenesis
- Pathology
  - ○ Substantia nigra (zona compacta) and locus ceruleus marked by loss of pigmented neurons
  - ○ Phagocytic cells with pigment
  - ○ Astrocytosis
  - ○ Lewy body—eosinophilic, cytoplasmic inclusion (intermediate filaments), 8–30 μm in diameter, may have a clear halo around it, present in 20% of normal people by age 80 yr, may be seen in Alzheimer's disease, stain with ubiquitin and α-synuclein
- Diffuse Lewy body disease
  - ○ May be on a continuum with Parkinson's disease
  - ○ Numerous widespread neocortical Lewy bodies (especially superior temporal lobe, cingulate gyrus, insular cortex layers V and VI)
  - ○ Often the neocortical Lewy bodies have atypical morphologies—ubiquitin stain maybe useful in highlighting their presence
  - ○ Many also have features of Alzheimer's disease
  - ○ More acute onset of symptoms/dementia, younger age of onset
- Postencephalitic Parkinson's disease
  - ○ Months or years after influenza pandemic of 1914–1918
  - ○ Loss of pigmented neurons, astrocytosis
  - ○ Neurofibrillary tangles, binucleated neurons

○ Few, if any, Lewy bodies

D. Parkinsonism–dementia complex of Guam

- Chamorro natives of Guam and Marina Islands
- Rigidity, bradykinesia, dementia
- Onset age 50–60 yr
- Death in 5 yr
- Generalized cerebral atrophy
- Tangles, neuron loss; no plaques, Lewy bodies, or inflammatory reaction
- Hippocampus, amygdaloid nucleus, temporal and frontal cortex, basal ganglia, substantia nigra
- Anterior horn cell disease in some patients (amyotrophic lateral sclerosis-like picture)—longer clinical course

E. Progressive supranuclear palsy

- AKA: Steele-Richardson-Olszewski syndrome
- Ophthalmoplegia (loss of vertical gaze), ataxia, expressionless facies, rigidity (hyperextension of head—posterior cervical muscle), mental disorders/dementia
- Onset 5th–7th decades
- Pathology
  - ○ Neuronal loss with tau positive tangles (straight filaments with a diameter of 15 nm), gliosis, and neuropil threads
  - ○ Basal ganglia and brain stem (substantia nigra, subthalamic nucleus, superior colliculi, periaqueductal gray, pontine tegmentum, dentate) the most severely involved areas, may see atrophy in these regions
  - ○ Astrocytes may also stain with tau protein

F. Hallervorden-Spatz disease

- Autosomal recessive
- Early childhood onset
- Dystonic posturing, choreoathetotic or tremulous movements, muscular rigidity and spasticity, dementia
- Death in 10–12 yr
- Pathology
  - ○ Rust brown discoloration of globus pallidus and substantia nigra
  - ○ Mineralization (iron) of vessel walls

○ Neuronal loss, axonal swelling

○ Demyelination

○ Astrocytosis

G. Striatonigral degeneration

- Clinically similar to Parkinson's disease
- Resistant to levodopa
- Atrophy of caudate, putamen, zona compacta of substantia nigra
- Neuron loss, astrocytosis
- No Lewy bodies, no tangles
- Cytoplasmic inclusions (tubular structures) in oligodendroglia and some neurons, nuclear inclusions in neurons and glial cells, neuropil threads—these findings also noted in Shy-Drager syndrome and olivopontocerebellar atrophy
- Part of multisystem atrophy syndrome

H. Shy-Drager syndrome

- Autonomic system failure with parkinsonism
- Loss of intermediolateral column neurons
- Pathology variable—between Parkinson's disease and striatonigral degeneration
- Part of multisystem atrophy syndrome

I. Olivopontocerebellar atrophy

- Ataxia, eye and somatic movement abnormalities, dysarthria, rigidity
- Most autosomal dominant
- Gross atrophy of basis pontis
- Depletion of Purkinje cells, loss of neurons in inferior olives
- Variable degeneration of spinal cord long tracts and neuronal loss/gliosis in putamen and substantia nigra
- Part of multisystem atrophy syndrome

J. Corticobasal degeneration

- 6th–7th decade
- Apraxia, limb dystonia, akinesia, rigidity, impaired ocular movement, dementia
- Frontoparietal atrophy
- Ballooned neurons
- Degeneration of subcortical nuclei, especially substantia nigra
- Neuronal inclusions (neurofibrillary tangle-like)—tau positive; ubiquitin positive

K. Friedreich's ataxia

- Familial form, onset 1st two decades
- Autosomal recessive
- Chromosome 9q13 (frataxin gene)
- GAA trinucleotide repeat expansion
- Ataxia, sensory disturbances (lower part of body—loss of joint position sense, vibration sense, two-point discrimination)
- Other neurologic disturbances—dysarthria, optic atrophy, deafness, dementia, epilepsy
- Skeletal deformities—pes cavus, kyphoscoliosis
- Heart abnormal—enlarged, pericardial adhesions, myocarditis
- Peak age of onset 10 yr
- Duration of disease 5–50 yr
- Death most commonly in 3rd and 4th decades (heart disease)
- Degeneration of sensory fibers, posterior roots, and ganglion cells in lower segment of cord
- Posterior column degeneration, gracilis > cuneatus
- Degeneration of dorsal nuclei (Clarke's column) and posterior > anterior spinocerebellar tract
- Cranial nerve tracts variably involved
- Cerebellar afferents (accessory cuneate nucleus) and outflow from dentate nucleus also involved

L. Dentorubropallidoluysial atrophy

- CAG trinucleotide repeat expansion
- Chromosome 12p
- Ataxia, chorea, myoclonic epilepsy, dementia
- Severe neuronal loss and gliosis in dentate nucleus, globus pallidus, red nucleus, and subthalamic nucleus
- Atrophy of superior cerebellar peduncles

M. Amyotrophic lateral sclerosis

- Male : Female 1.7 : 1
- Middle-aged and elderly
- 5-10% familial autosomal dominant, genetic locus for some of this group on SOD1 gene on chromosome 21q
- Weakness and pain—in extremities or bulbar musculature

- Asymmetrical → symmetrical extremity involvement
- Muscle wasting, fasciculation, sensation intact
- CSF normal
- 2–3 yr to death
- Cause of death—respiratory failure and pneumonia
- Atrophy of anterior spinal nerve roots and affected muscles
- Precentral gyrus atrophic
- Loss of anterior horn cells (lumbar, cervical cord)
- Several types of inclusions may be seen in motor neurons
  - Bunina bodies—small eosinophilic inclusions (2–5 μm)
  - Hyaline inclusions
  - Basophilic large inclusions
  - Aggregates of thread-like structures called skeins (seen on ubiquitin staining)
- Neuronal loss of hypoglossal nuclei and other cranial nerve nuclei (facial, trigeminal)
- Pyramidal tract degeneration
- Neuronophagia and gliosis

N. Spinal muscular atrophies

- Variety of types
  - Werdnig-Hoffmann—prototypical
  - Kugelberg-Welander
  - Adult onset forms
  - Later onset—more favorable prognosis
- Werdnig-Hoffman disease
  - Autosomal recessive
  - Chromosome 5q11–13
  - 1 : 20,000
  - Death before 2 yr
  - Proximal > distal onset of weakness
  - Hypotonia, "floppy baby"
  - Decreased fetal movement—3rd trimester
  - Facial muscles spared
  - Fasciculations of tongue
  - Loss of anterior horn cell neurons of spinal cord

- Atrophy of anterior spinal roots

- Neurogenic muscle disease—rounded fiber atrophy

- Loss of neurons in nuclei ambigui, hypoglossal and facial nuclei

- Onuf's nucleus spared

9 CNS Infection

I. General Information
  A. CNS protection
    - CSF lacks host defense
    - Meninges
    - Blood-brain barrier
  B. Routes of infection
    - Direct implantation
    - Shunt
    - Local spread
    - Hematogenous
    - Septic emboli
  C. Factors in infection
    - Number of organisms
    - Host immune system
    - Type of organism
  D. Pathophysiology of infection
    - Injury to blood-brain barrier
    - Separation of tight junctions
    - Increased albumin in CSF, increased ICP
    - Edema (vasogenic and inflammatory mediators)
    - Spinal nerve root and nerve (neck stiffness)
    - Vasculitis; infarction
    - Direct cytopathic/toxic effect
II. Suppurative Lesions
  A. Epidural abscess
    - Extension from bones (trauma, osteomyelitis, otitis)
    - Less often extension from soft tissue (venous)
    - Associated with prior surgery or trauma
    - Most common organisms are Streptococcus followed by Staphylococcus
    - Intracranial
      ○ Most often related to extension from a frontal or mastoid sinus infection or focus of osteomyelitis
      ○ Circumscribed, flattened
      ○ Adhesion of dura to bone confines abscess
      ○ May cause subdural abscess, leptomeningitis
    - Spinal
      ○ Thoracic and lumbar regions
      ○ More common than intracranial epidural abscesses
      ○ Compression of cord and roots
      ○ Staphylococcus aureus
  B. Subdural abscess
    - Secondary to bone/sinus infection (especially paranasal sinuses, middle ear, cranium) via thrombophlebitis
    - Dorsolateral aspect of cerebrum, frontal polar region, interhemispheric fissure
    - Adhesions, loculation
    - Compression of brain, increased ICP
    - Streptococcus (#1) and Staphylococcus (#2)
    - Spinal subdural rare
  C. Leptomeningitis
    - Neutrophils, fibrin in the leptomeninges

- With treatment, the inflammatory infiltrate may switch to more lymphocytes, macrophages, and plasma cells
- Arterial subintimal infiltration
- Thrombosis, vasculitis, infarct, hemorrhage, cerebral edema, vascular congestion
- Virchow-Robin space extension
- May extend to cause ependymitis, ventriculitis
- Subarachnoid fibrosis, CSF obstruction, subependymal gliosis with healing
- Neonatal (maternal genital flora)—community acquired
  - *Strep. agalactiae* (group B)—exudate over vertex
  - *E. coli*—hemorrhage, necrotizing arteritis, necrosis, roughly same incidence in this age group as *Strep. agalactiae*
  - Proteus
  - *Listeria*—microabscesses
- Childhood—community acquired
  - *Neisseria meningitidis*—basal, young adults, army recruits, most epidemic outbreaks related to group A, associated with Waterhouse-Friderichsen syndrome [dissoninated intravascular coagulopathy (DIC) picture with hemorrhagic adrenal glands]
  - *H. influenza*—vertex, cortical softening, venous thrombosis
  - *Strep. pneumoniae*—vertex
- Adults/elderly—community acquired
  - *Strep. pneumoniae*
  - *Listeria*
  - Any organism is possible with hospital-acquired infections

D. Abscess
- Localized suppuration within brain substance
- Streptococcus (#1), Gram-negative bacilli (#2) Staphylococcus (#3), may see anaerobes and aerobes
- Frequently multiple organisms
- Focal septic encephalitis (cerebritis), peripheral edema
- Early: central—pus; middle—granulation tissue; outer—astrocytosis/edema
- Later: central—liquefaction; middle—collagenous wall; outer—astrocytosis
- Granulation tissue—contrast enhances on CT scan as a result of hypervascularity
- Hematogenous (metastatic) abscesses—often multiple
- Damage a result of local tissue destruction, edema (mass effect)
- Consequences
  - Organization
  - Formation of daughter abscess
  - Ependymitis
  - Leptomeningitis

E. Septic embolism
- Occlusion—infarction
- Infection—arteritis, septic aneurysm, hemorrhage, septic infarcts
- Small parenchymal arteries—microabscess, petechiae
- Septicemia—capillaries, microabscess
- Leptomeninges—septic infarct, hemorrhage, meningitis
- Large artery—infarct
- Trunk artery base of brain—subarachnoid bleed

F. Tuberculosis (TB)
- Epidural
  - Extension from vertebral infection (Pott's disease)
  - Compression of cord
  - Rarely causes meningitis
- Subdural
  - Miliary or tuberculoma-en-plaque
- Tuberculoma = abscess
- Granulomas with caseous necrosis
- Usually small and multiple
- May act as mass
- Enhancing on CT scan
- TB meningitis—base of brain; neutrophils, fibrin, endarteritis, hemorrhage, caseous necrosis, granulomatous inflammation.
- CSF studies: lymphocyte predominance with

pleocytosis, elevated protein, decreased glucose

- Culture still remains gold standard for diagnosis, molecular biologic techniques exist to identify the organisms
- Use of special stains (such as Ziehl-Neelsen, fite) on tissue sections has a relatively low yield (<50%)
- Other nontuberculous mycobacteria may infect CNS
  - Mycobacterium avium intracellulare typically marked by perivascular macrophages with organism; rarely presents as a tumor-like nodule with fibrosis

G. Sarcoidosis

- Noncaseating granulomas
- Base of brain, posterior fossa
- Near vessels in meninges
- Optic nerve and chiasm involvement common
- Course usually slow, may be rapidly fatal
- Hydrocephalus, cranial nerve defects, hypothalamic symptoms
- May have no apparent systemic disease

H. Whipple's disesase

- Caused by *Tropheryma whippelii*, a Gram-positive actinomycete
- PAS-positive organisms in macrophages that are often arranged in perivascular distribution

I. Syphilis

- Caused by *Treponema pallidum*
- Highlighted with special stains (e.g., Steiner, Warthin-Starry, Dieterle)
- Subacute secondary lymphocytic meningitis
- Meningovascular
  - Lymphs, plasma cells ± gummata (central necrosis surrounded by epithelioid histiocytes, fibroblasts, and multinucleated giant cells)
  - Do not usually see organisms with gumma because it represents a hyperimmune form of tissue necrosis
  - Perivascular parenchymal inflammation
  - Arteritis, intimal proliferation, Heubner's endarteritis obliterans (collagenous thick-

ening of the intima and thinning of the media), which may lead to infarct
  - Pachymeningitis cervicalis hypertrophicans—cervical fibrosis of dura to pia
- General paresis
  - Brain invasion—subacute encephalitis
  - Prolonged secondary stage—failure to produce neutralizing/destructive antibody or failure of antibody to reach spirochete
  - Early—brain grossly normal
  - Later—frontal atrophy
  - Loss of neurons, astrocytosis, capillary proliferation, perivascular inflammation, microglia with iron
  - Spirochetes may be hard to identify, 3-yr course
- Lissauer's dementia
  - Variant of general paresis
  - Epileptic or apoplectiform attacks
  - Focal signs
  - Average 7 to 8-yr course
  - Temporal atrophy with pseudolaminar degeneration
- Tabes dorsalis
  - Degeneration of spinal dorsal roots and columns
  - Lumbosacral and lower thoracic cord
  - Dorsal root ganglia unaffected
  - May see meningovascular disease
- Optic atrophy
  - Chronic pial inflammation, degeneration of nerve
  - Peripheral > central
  - Associated with tabes dorsalis
- Congenital
  - Meningovascular with obstruction, hydrocephalus
  - General paresis—especially cerebellum
  - Rarely tabes dorsalis

J. Lyme disease

- Caused by *Borrelia burgdorferi* (a spirochete transmitted by ioxodid ticks)

- Associated skin lesions (erythema chronicum migrans)
- Lymphoplasmacytic leptomeningitis

III. Fungal Infection

  A. General

- Immunocompromised persons at risk
- Secondary spread common
- Hematogenous spread > contiguous spread
- Granulomatous inflammation and abscess are common patterns of injury
- Septic emboli, may result in mycotic aneurysm

  B. Cryptococcosis

- Budding yeast, thick mucopolysaccharide wall
- Pigeon excrement
- Entry—pulmonary > skin
- Pathology
  - Leptomeningitis, gelatinous "bubbly" exudate
  - Macrophages
  - Perivascular extension, may be quite extensive and give the brain a honeycomb look grossly
  - Granulomas, "torulomas" (abscesses)
  - Organisms highlighted with PAS, mucicarmine stains

  C. Candidiasis

- Budding cells, branching pseudohyphae
- Entry—skin, GI tract
- CNS disease as a result of systemic infection or endocarditis
- Pathology
  - Chronic granulomas
  - Microabscesses
  - Rarely arteritis, basal leptomeningitis
  - Organisms highlighted on Gomori methenamine silver (GMS) or PAS stains

  D. Aspergillosis

- Dichotomously branching septate hyphae
- Entry—airborne lung infection followed by hematogenous spread, may also get disseminated from other organ system involvement

or rarely direct extension from an orbital or paranasal sinus infection

- Pathology
  - Granuloma—abscess ± basal meningitis
  - Septic infarcts secondary to vascular infiltration, hemorrhage
  - Focal cerebritis, especially white matter

  E. Mucormycosis

- Broad branching, nonseptate hyphae (10–15 μm)
- Genera of Mucoraceae family, including Rhizopus, Absidia, Mucor, Rhizomucor, Apophysomyces, and Chlamydoabsidia
- Entry—nasal sinus, extension into orbit, aspiration into lung
- Pathology
  - Acute meningeal inflammation
  - Hemorrhagic coagulative necrosis of brain (ventral)
  - Vascular luminal and mural invasion

  F. Coccidioidomycosis

- Semiarid areas (South America and southwest United States)
- Double-contoured, refractile capsules with endospores
- Self-limited respiratory infection
- 0.05% cases disseminate, CNS disease in 10–25% of these cases
- Pathology
  - Basilar meningitis—neutrophils, fibrinous exudate
  - Later—granulomas, fibrosis
  - Cranial osteomyelitis
  - Parenchymal granulomas rare

  G. Blastomycosis

- Males > females, agricultural workers
- Acquired from contaminated soil, southeastern United States
- Broad-based budding
- Protoplasmic body (10–15 μm in diameter)
- No hyphae in tissue sections
- Lung and skin entry portals
- Leptomeningitis and granulomas rare, often presents as abscess

H. Histoplasmosis
- Entry—inhalation of dust containing spores
- *Histoplasma capsulatum* consists of small ovoid and budding bodies, PAS and GMS positive
- Only rarely disseminates to involve the CNS
- Necrosis with macrophages (containing organisms), lymphocytes, and plasma cells

I. Actinomycosis
- Bacteria with fungal-like morphology
- Thin (<1 μm pseudohyphae) filaments
- Gram-positive, acid-fast negative
- Sulfur granules
- Entry—cervicofacial
- Pathology
  - Granuloma—abscess, multiple
  - Basilar meningitis

J. Nocardiosis
- Bacteria with fungal-like morphology
- Thin filaments
- Gram-positive, partial acid-fast positive
- No sulfur granules
- Entry—lung
- Pathology
  - Granulomas, small and mulitple

IV. Viral Infection
A. General
- Routes of spread
  - Hematogenous (polio, arbovirus)
  - Peripheral nerve (rabies)
  - Olfactory mucosa, trigeminal nerve (herpes)
- Morphologic features
  - Little (edema, congestion) or no distinctive gross alterations (except herpes, progressive multifocal leukoencephalopathy [PML])
  - Diffuse distribution (except polio, herpes zoster)
  - Primary neuronal involvement common
- Common histopathologic features
  - Nerve cell alterations
    - Degeneration—chromatolysis, eosinophilia, nuclear changes, neuronophagia
    - Eosinophilic nuclear inclusions (Cowdry)
      - Type A—intranuclear, large spherical, halo (e.g., CMV, herpes, PML)
      - Type B—small, multiple, no nucleolar displacement (e.g., polio)
      - Intracytoplasmic
  - Reactive endothelial changes
  - Tissue necrosis or demyelination with certain viruses
  - Inflammatory cell exudate
    - Microglia—diffuse or focal (neuronophagia, glial nodule, glial shrub, glial scar)
    - Chronic inflammatory cells (lymphocytes, plasma cells and macrophages), often perivascular distribution

B. Polio
- Acute febrile disease, asymmetric paralysis (legs > arms > trunk)
- 5% mortality
- Pathology
  - Large motor neurons lost (anterior horn cells, motor neurons of cranial nerves)
  - Lymphocytic perivascular and meningeal inflammation
  - Gliosis and microgliosis with recovery

C. Arbovirus
- Arthropod (RNA viruses)—mosquito borne
- Serologic exam to make diagnosis
- In United States—St Louis, California virus, Eastern and Western Equine encephalitis
- Pathology
  - Brain congestion and edema
  - Widespread, gray matter
  - Most severe changes with Eastern equine
  - Neuronal degeneration, microglial nodules, perivascular and meningeal chronic inflammation; abscess and neutrophils in severe cases

D. "Aseptic Meningitis"
- Refers to any culture-negative meningitis
- Many viruses—Coxsackie and Echovirus most cases

- Low mortality
- Meningeal and choroid plexus lymphs

E. Influenza
- Onset respiratory
- Abnormal behavior, disoriented, seizures, coma
- Neuronal degeneration, inflammation

F. Measles
- Mostly < age 10 yr
- Low fatality
- Perivascular inflammation, demyelination
- Multinucleated giant cells, intranuclear and intracytoplasmic inclusions

G. Subacute sclerosing panencephalitis (SSPE)
- Fatal, measles virus
- Under age 12 yr
- Course: months to a few years
- Progressive dementia, myoclonus, seizures, ataxia, dystonia
- Pathology
  - Gray matter subacute encephalitis
  - Eosinophilic nuclear and cytoplasmic inclusions, neuronal loss, microglial proliferation, perivascular inflammation
  - Demyelination, oligodendroglial inclusions, reactive astrocytosis
  - Cerebral atrophy—old cases
  - May see occasional neurofibrillary tangles

H. Mumps
- 2–10 d after onset
- Low mortality
- Perivenous demyelination
- 10–20% aseptic meningitis

I. Rabies
- Variable incubation (1–3 mo)
- Bite of infected animal—skunk, racoon, etc.
- Anxiety, psychomotor sensitivity, hydrophobia, dysphagia, seizures
- Death 2–7 d
- Pathology
  - Encephalomyelitis (especially brain stem)
  - Glial nodules
  - Negri bodies (hippocampus, cerebel-

lum)—eosinophilic cytoplasmic neuronal inclusion with basophilic inner formation
  - Lyssa body—lack inner formation

J. Herpes simplex
- 70% fatal
- No seasonal incidence
- May see no obvious skin or visceral disease, the virus often replicates at a peripheral site before reaching the CNS
- Virus often later peripherally located and may be reactivated by a variety of factors (stress, fever, sunlight, trauma, radiation)
- Virus spreads from periphery to ganglion via retrograde axoplasmic transport
- Pathology
  - Congenital—acute encephalitis with visceral lesion, herpes type I
  - Adults—herpes type II, acute hemorrhagic necrotizing encephalitis (basal frontal, cingulate, temporal gyri, insula)
  - Eosinophilic nuclear inclusions in glial cells (oligodendrocytes > astrocytes)

K. Herpes zoster
- Skin lesions (shingles)—vesicles in a sensory nerve dermatome distribution
- Acute cerebellar disease—nystagmus, dysarthria, ataxia
- Pathology
  - Dorsal ganglia—inflammation, petechiae, degenerating neurons
  - Eosinophilic intranuclear inclusions
  - Meningeal inflammation, granulomatous angiitis

L. Cytomegalovirus
- Infant—transplacental transmission, stillbirth, prematurity
- Adult—rare, less extensive, immunocompromised states (18–33% of AIDS patients have evidence of CMV in brain)
- Pathology
  - Infants—necrosis, inclusions (neurons, glial cells, endothelial cells), chorioretinitis; endstage—gliosis, calcification, hydrocephalus, microcephaly
  - Adults—microglial aggregates

- Large cells with intranuclear (Cowdry A) and cytoplasmic inclusions

- May involve ependyma and subependymal regions (hemorrhagic necrotizing ventriculoencephalitis and choroid plexitis)

M. Progressive multifocal leukoencephalopathy (PML)

- Immunocompromised states

- Progressive disturbances in motor and mental function and vision

- Papova virus (JC, SV40)—DNA virus

- Demyelination—multifocal, asymmetric

- Astrocytosis

- Alzheimer I astrocytes—bizarre, atypical astrocytes; probable viral cytopathic effect

- Intranuclear inclusions—oligodendrocytes (Cowdry A)

- Paucity of lymphocytes

N. HIV

- RNA retrovirus

- 10% develop "aseptic" meningitis within 1–2 wk of seroconversion

- Meningoencephalitis often presents with dementia, seizures, myoclonus and focal motor signs

- Chronic inflammation with microglial nodules

- Microglial nodules often contain macrophage-derived multinucleated giant cells

- Virus can be detected in macrophages, CD4-positive lymphs and microglia

- Areas most severely affected include deep cerebral white matter, basal ganglia, cerebral cortex, and brain stem

- Vacuolar myelopathy involving degeneration of spinal cord (worst in thoracic cord), especially posterior columns; presents as progressive paraparesis, sensory ataxia, and incontinence; swelling between myelin sheaths, reactive astrocytosis, macrophage infiltrate and occasional multinucleated giant cells.

- AIDS in children frequently marked by calcification of parenchymal vessels within basal ganglia and deep cerebral white matter

- At risk for opportunistic infections

O. Human T lymphotropic virus type 1 (HTLV-1)

- Retrovirus causing tropical spastic paraparesis

- Myelin loss and axonal degeneration in spinal cord white matter, leptomeningeal chronic inflammation and fibrosis, gliosis

- Thoracic and lumbar regions particularly susceptible

- May see demyelination of optic and auditory nerves

V. Parasitic Infections

A. Toxoplasmosis

- Caused by *Toxoplasma gondii* infection

- Congenital form

- Occurs only if the maternal infection is acquired during pregnancy

- Miliary granulomata

- Necrosis

- Calcification

- Meningitis, chorioretinitis

- Adult

- May rarely encounter cysts in an incompetent individual

- Space-occupying lesion(s)—abscesses, may demonstrate the same architectural features of a bacterial abscess

- Scattered necrotic foci

- Rarely microglial nodules/encephalitis picture

B. Amebiasis

- *Entamoeba histolytica* or *Iodamoeba buetschlii*

- Naegleria—via nasal cavity, often acquired by swimming in contaminated water, purulent meningitis, rapidly progressive, severe involvement of the olfactory area (often the point of entry)

- Acanthamoeba—diffuse necrotizing granulomatous encephalitis and meningitis

- Often see trophozoites in tissue section

C. Malaria

- 2% of cases of *Plasmodium falciparum*

- Presents with headache, drowsiness, confusion, coma, fevers

- Often see the organisms in peripheral blood

- Grossly, see opacity of meninges, dusky coloration of the gray matter, edema, congestion
- Capillaries filled with organism
- Small foci of ischemic necrosis rimmed by microglia (Dürcks nodes)
- White matter petechiae
- Can see granules of dark malarial pigment in red cells

D. Cysticercosis
- *Taenia solium* (pork tapeworm)
- Larvae encysts in brain
- Inflammation, granuloma, calcification

E. Schistosomiasis
- *S. japonicum*—cerebrum lesions
- *S. mansoni, S. hematobium*—spinal cord lesions
- Necrotizing inflammation with neutrophils, eosinophils, giant cells
- Fibrosis and calcification with healing

F. Trypanosomiasis
- African disease caused by *T. brucei*; acquired by bite of tsetse fly; may present with fever, rash, edema, cardiac involvement, anemia; meningoencephalitis occurs during late stages of the disease
- South American disease (Chagas disease) caused by *T. cruzi*; acquired from feces of the reduviid bug; brain with edema, congestion, hemorrhages, microglial nodules, granulomas

G. A variety of other parasites have been described to cause CNS pathology, including Echinococcus, Spirometria (Spanganosis), Paragonimus (lung fluke), Trichinella spiralis, Loa Loa, Onchocerca, and Strongyloides

VI. Transmissible Spongiform Encephalopathies
A. General
- Includes Creutzfeldt-Jakob disease, Gerstmann-Straussler-Scheinker, Kuru, familial insomia
- Related to prion protein abnormalties
- Prion protein is a normal 30 Kd cellular protein present in neurons (chromosome 20)
- In disease, protein undergoes conformational change from normal α-helix isoform to an abnormal β-pleated sheet isoform (PrP^{sc} or PrP^{res})

- Conformational change promotes further production of the abnormal prion protein material
- Prion protein inactivated by autoclaving or bleach

B. Creutzfeldt-Jakob disease (CJD)
- $1/10^6$ incidence
- Subacute dementia
- Myoclonus
- EEG—biphasic, triphasic spikes
- Onset > 30 yr; female : male 2 : 1
- Duration < 1 yr
- Can evaluate CSF for 14-3-3 protein to support diagnosis
- Pathology
  - Spongiform change
  - Neuronal atrophy/loss
  - Gliosis
  - Granular layer degeneration
  - Kuru plaque 10% (extracellular deposits of aggregated abnormal protein—Congo red and PAS positive), prominent in variant CJD, which may be related to ingestion of contaminated beef (mad cow disease)
  - Iatrogenic transmission documented (e.g., pooled pituitary hormone preparations, dura mater and corneal grafts/transplants)

C. Gerstmann-Straussler-Scheinker disease
- Ataxia
- Behavioral change
- Late dementia
- Autosomal dominant, onset > 30 yr
- Duration—5 yr
- 1/10 million incidence
- Corticospinal tract degeneration
- No/mild spongiform change and astrocytosis
- Cerebellar plaques

D. Kuru
- Cannibalism: Papua New Guinea; Fore tribe—women and children
- Tremor, ataxia, dysphagia, euphoria
- Duration of disease < 1 yr
- Severe cerebellum disease—kuru plaques, axon torpedoes, granular layer degeneration

E. Familial insomnia

- Sleep disorder, bizarre behavior, autonomic dysfunction

- Adult onset, autosomal dominant

- Duration of disease < 2 yr

- Severe anterior and medial thalamus gliosis, inferior olive degeneration

10 Skeletal Muscle

I. General Information

  A. Muscle biopsy

- Do not biopsy muscle with needle in it (EMG), injection site (gluteus, deltoid), severely diseased muscle
- Commonly biopsied muscles: quadriceps (vastus lateralis), triceps, biceps, and gastrocnemius

  B. Clinical information useful when interpreting a muscle biopsy

- Age
- Gender
- Drugs/medications
- Medical/family history
- EMG findings

  C. A variety of enzyme histochemical stains and special stains are used in the evaluation of biopsy specimens. Many of these stains require fresh or frozen tissue to work. Improper freezing of the specimen may result in a vacuolar artifact.

  D. Staining of the muscle biopsy specimen

- Routine hematoxylin and eosin
- Acid phosphatase
  - Lysosomal enzyme
  - Increased with degeneration (red staining)
  - Inflammatory cells
- Alkaline phosphatase
  - Normal capillary basement stains
  - Regenerating fibers (black staining)
- Trichrome (Gomori)
  - Nuclei red
  - Ragged red fibers (mitochondria)
  - Inclusion body myositis inclusion (rimmed vacuoles)
  - Fibrosis
- PAS
  - Normal muscle with glycogen
  - Type I > type II
  - Glycogen storage diseases
- Oil-Red-O
  - Normally evenly distributed
  - Type I > type II
  - Lipid disorders
- (SAB) Sulfonated alcian blue/Congo red
  - Amyloid
  - Mast cells (SAB positive—internal control)
- Nonspecific esterase
  - Angular atrophic fibers (neurogenic)
  - Acetylcholinesterase
  - Type I > type II
  - Acute denervation (6 mo)
  - Some inflammatory cells
- NADH
  - Oxidative enzyme
  - Type I > type II

- ○ Myofibrillary network inside muscle fiber
- Cytochrome oxidase
  - ○ Mitochondrial enzyme
  - ○ Type I > type II
  - ○ Focal deficiencies exist
- ATPase (adenosine triphosphatase)
  - ○ pH 4.6 (reverse) or pH 4.3
    - ▸ Type I dark
    - ▸ Type IIA light
    - ▸ Type IIB intermediate
    - ▸ Type IIC light (pH 4.2)
  - ○ pH 9.8 (standard)
    - ▸ Type I light
    - ▸ Type II dark
- Succinate dehydrogenase (SDH)
  - ○ Mitochondrial enzyme
  - ○ Type I > type II
- A variety of other stains may be selectively performed including myophosphorylase, myoadenylate deaminase, phosphofructokinase, etc.

E. Tissue is often processed in glutaraldehyde or other fixative for potential electron microscopic evaluation

F. In cases of suspected metabolic disease, extra frozen tissue for assay purposes is warranted.

II. Myopathic Versus Neurogenic Changes

A. Myopathic processes include such disease entities as inflammatory myopathies, muscular dystrophies, congenital myopathies and metabolic diseases

B. Myopathic changes
- Irregularity of fiber size
- Rounded fibers
- Centralized nuclei
- Necrotic and basophilic fibers
- Cytoplasmic alterations
- Interstitial fibrosis
- Absence of enzyme staining
- Inflammation
- Storage of glycogen and lipid

C. Neurogenic diseases include those processes that affect the peripheral/central nervous sys-

tem and result in secondary changes in the muscle

D. Neurogenic changes
- Angular atrophic fibers (esterase positive)
- Group atrophy
- Fiber type grouping
- Target and targetoid fibers
- Nuclear bags
- No necrotic or basophilic fibers
- Minimal interstitial fibrosis
- No inflammation
- No centralized nuclei

III. Inflammatory Myopathies

A. Polymyositis
- 30–60% of inflammatory myopathies
- Nonhereditary
- Adults (age 40–60 yr), second peak in childhood
- Male : female 1 : 2
- Idiopathic versus connective tissue disease (SLE, rheumatoid arthritis associated)
- An association with neoplasms in adults
- Proximal muscle weakness, often painful
- Fatigue, fever, weight loss
- CPK and aldolase elevated
- Most respond to steroids or other immunosuppressives
- EMG—fibrillation potential in acute stage, polyphasic short duration potentials
- Histopathology
  - ○ Increased variation of myofiber size, central nuclei
  - ○ Inflammation (lymphocytes and macrophages), endomysial (surrounding individual muscle fibers)
  - ○ CD4-positive lymphocytes more common around vessels
  - ○ CD8-positive lymphocytes more common in endomysium
  - ○ Degeneration
  - ○ Regeneration—basophilic staining cytoplasm, nuclear enlargement with prominent nucleolus
  - ○ Vasculitis (lymphocytic, nonnecrotizing)

     ◦ Endomysial fibrosis

     ◦ Motheaten fibers

        ▶ Ill-defined zones of enzyme loss

        ▶ Type I > type II

        ▶ Nonspecific findings in myopathies

B. Dermatomyositis

- Proximal muscle weakness

- Heliotropic rash, Gottron's papules

- Dysphagia, arthralgias, constitutional symptoms

- Childhood disease often associated with vasculitis and calcinosis, not associated with malignancy

- Associated with connective tissue disease

- Associated with malignancy in 7–30% of cases, elderly patients (>55–60 yr); cancers of the breast, ovary, lung, prostate, colon

- Histopathology

     ◦ Inflammation—perivascular, may be scant, mixture of T- and B-lymphocytes (vasculopathic disease)

     ◦ May see non-necrotizing lymphocytic vasculitis, thrombosis

     ◦ Degeneration

     ◦ Regeneration

     ◦ Perifascicular atrophy—ischemia related

C. Inclusion body myositis

- Most > 50 yr, males > females

- Progressive, painless muscle weakness

- Steroid resistant

- Enzymes sometimes normal

- EMG—neurogenic picture

- Etiology not known

- Tubulofilaments (15–18 nm) on electron microscopy, most readily found in fibers with rimmed vacuoles

- May see amyloid protein material

- Mitochondrial abnormalities frequent concommitant finding

- Histopathology

     ◦ Inflammation

     ◦ Degeneration

     ◦ Regeneration

     ◦ Rimmed vacuoles—autophagic vacuoles, granular basophilic material on trichrome stain

     ◦ Rare intranuclear inclusions

     ◦ Frequent neurogenic atrophy-like component

D. Rheumatoid arthritis

- Type II atrophy

- Moth-eaten fibers common

- Severe disease—type I and type II atrophy, ring fibers, increased central nuclei

- Chronic inflammation, either polymyositis or focal nodular myositis pattern of injury

- Vasculitis—usually non-necrotizing lymphocytic

E. Bacterial myositis

- Often related to skin injury

- Gas gangrene (Clostridium)

- Pyomyositis (Staph)

- Neutrophils frequently present

F. Viral myositis

- Muscle pain and muscle weakness usually not salient features

- Influenza A and B

- Enterovirus

- HIV (AZT treatment)—AZT may also result in mitochondrial abnormality

- Coxsackie B (epidemic pleurodynia, Bornholm's disease)

G. Parasitic myositis

- Trichinosis (*Trichinella spiralis*)

     ◦ Encysted larvae

     ◦ Granulomatous inflammation with eosinophils

     ◦ Inadequately cooked meat

- Toxocariasis, Cysticercosis, Hydatidosis, Toxoplasmosis, Sarcosporidiosis, Trypanosomiasis

H. Fungal myositis

- Very rare

- Candida and cryptococcus the most common

I. Vasculitis

- May see vasculitic component to another inflammatory myopathic process (generally non-necrotizing lymphocytic vasculitis) or may be part of systemic vasculitis process such as polyarteritis nodosa

- Polyarteritis nodosa (PAN) affects medium to small size arterial vessels causing fibrinoid necrosis of vessel walls
- With PAN, will often see vessels at various stages of the disease process in the same biopsy
- May be associated with denervation atrophy changes (presumably related to involvement of peripheral nerves)

IV. Denervation Atrophy

A. General information

- Group of disorders that affect anterior horn cells, nerve roots, or peripheral nerves causing secondary changes in the skeletal muscle
- Types of neurogenic disease
  - ○ Motor neuron
    - ▶ Amyotropic lateral sclerosis (ALS)
    - ▶ Spinal muscular atrophy (Werdnig-Hoffmann, Kugelberg-Welander)
  - ○ Motor endplate
    - ▶ Myasthenia gravis
  - ○ Peripheral (motor) neuropathy
  - ○ Metabolic
  - ○ Toxic
  - ○ Vascular/connective tissue disease
  - ○ Systemic disease (diabetes, uremia)
  - ○ Infection
  - ○ Malignancies
- Histopathology
  - ○ Angulated fiber atrophy (esterase positive)
  - ○ Type I and type II fibers both involved
  - ○ Increased NADH staining in angular atrophic fibers
  - ○ Nest-like fascicular atrophy—two contiguous motor units involved
  - ○ Nuclear bags—endstage
  - ○ May see evidence of reinnervation
    - ▶ Collateral sprouting of spared motor neurons

- ▶ Type grouping—10 fibers of the same type contiguous along 1 edge
- ▶ Target fibers
  - ▷ Type I > type II fibers
  - ▷ Three zones of staining: central pale zone devoid of oxidative activity; dark annular intermediate zone rich in oxidative enzymes; normal peripheral zone
  - ▷ Targetoid fibers (core fibers)—no intermediate zone, type II predilection, a less specific finding

B. Spinal muscular atrophies

- Includes those disorders that cause anterior horn cell degeneration such as Werdnig-Hoffman disease, Kugelberg-Welander disease, etc. (*see* Neurodegenerative diseases)
- Chromosome 5 (survival motor neuron gene)
- EMG findings confirm denervation
- CPK levels often normal or slightly elevated
- Fascicular atrophy, rounded fiber atrophy in infantile variant
- In later onset varients, see angular atrophic esterase positive fibers instead of rounded fiber atrophy
- Scattered type I hypertrophic fibers
- Increased endomysial fibrofatty tissue
- Increase in muscle spindle number

C. Myasthenia gravis

- Immune-mediated loss of acetylcholine receptors with circulating antibodies to acetylcholine receptor
- Prevalence of about 3/100,000 persons
- In young patients (<40 yr), women > men; in older patients, equal gender distribution
- Associated with thymic hyperplasia (65%) and thymoma (15%)
- Normal nerve conduction studies
- Decreasing motor response with repeated stimulation
- Presents with weakness of extraocular muscle, fluctuating generalized weakness
- Improved strength in response to acetylcholinesterase agents
- Histopathology

- ○ Type II atrophy
- ○ Ultrastructurally, may see simplification of the postsynaptic membrane
- ○ Lymphorrhages (lymphoid aggregates) in about 25% of cases
- ○ May see evidence of mild denervation atrophy

D. Lambert-Eaton myasthenic syndrome
- Usually develops as a paraneoplastic process (especially with small cell carcinoma of lung)
- Proximal muscle weakness with autonomic dysfunction
- Enhanced neurotransmission with repeated stimulation
- Decrease in the number of vesicles released in response to each presynaptic action potential
- Some patients with antibodies to presynaptic calcium channels

V. Congential Myopathies
A. General information
- Disorders of muscle fiber maturation and reorganization
- Nonprogressive/slowly progressive
- Retarded motor development, muscle weakness
- Frequently associated with skeletal dysmorphism
- May present as "floppy baby" due to hypotonia or with joint contractures (arthrogryposis)
- Familial incidence
- Specific structural abnormality of muscle fibers

B. Nemaline myopathy
- Weakness, hypotonia, and delayed motor development in childhood, may present in adulthood
- Autosomal recessive, autosomal dominant and sporadic variants recognized
- CPK often normal or mildly elevated
- Intracytoplasmic nemaline rodlets (red on trichrome)
- Number of affected fibers has no correlation with disease severity

- Both type I and type II fibers affected
- Nemaline rods not specific for nemaline myopathy—reported in a variety of other muscle disorders
- Rods derived from Z-band material (α-actinin)

C. Central core disease
- Early-onset hypotonia and nonprogressive muscle weakness
- Joint deformities such as hip dislocations common
- May develop malignant hyperthermia
- Autosomal dominant condition related to defect of ryanodine receptor-1 gene (chromosome 19q13.1)
- CPK generally normal or slightly elevated, especially in later-onset cases
- Cytoplasmic cores devoid of enzyme activity (NADH negative) in many fibers
- Cores may be eccentrically placed and multiple
- Cores generally confined to type I fibers
- Ultrastructurally, cores are zones in which myofilaments are densely packed with absence of mitochondria, glycogen, and lipids
- Minicore or multicore disease is a distinct autosomal recessive condition

D. Centronuclear (myotubular) myopathy
- Presents in infancy or childhood with involvement of extraocular and facial muscles, hypotonia, and slowly progressive limb muscle weakness
- CPK may be normal or slightly elevated
- X-linked autosomal recessive or sporadic variants
- Increased numbers of centrally placed nuclei (involving most myofibers)
- Most fibers containing central nuclei are type I and tend to be somewhat atrophic
- Small zones surrounding the nuclei that are devoid of myofibrils and filled with mitochondrial aggregates, lipid, and glycogen

E. Congenital fiber type disproportion
- Autosomal recessive condition
- Variable presentation clinically; hypotonia,

long thin face, contractures, congenital hip dislocation, respiratory problems

- Mean fiber diameter of type I fibers at least 12% smaller than type II fibers

- May also see increased numbers of centralized nuclei, moth-eaten fibers and nemaline rods

VI. Metabolic Myopathies

   A. Mitochondrial myopathy

   - Many related to mutations in either nuclear or mitochondrial genes

   - Three categories of genetic alterations

     ○ Class I mutations: involve nuclear DNA (e.g., Leigh's syndrome)

     ○ Class II mutations: point mutations of mitochondrial DNA (e.g., MERFF and MELAS)

     ○ Class III mutations: deletions or duplications of mitochondrial DNA (e.g., Kearns-Sayre syndrome)

   - May be related to abnormalities of mitochondrial transport, substrate utilization, Krebs cycle, oxidative—phosphorylation coupling, or the respiratory chain (the most common group of mitochondrial myopathies)

   - Myopathy only presentation in some patients

   - Cerebral dysfunction with myopathy in some patients (mitochondrial encephalomyopathies)

   - Progressive external ophthalmoplegia, proximal muscle weakness

   - Ragged red fibers (Gomori trichrome stain)—related to aggregates of often morphologically abnormal mitochondria situated in a subsarcolemmal location)

   - Not all myofibers equally affected

   - Often nonspecific increase in lipid and glycogen

   - Sporadic and inherited forms

   - Abnormal mitochondrial structure on electron microscopic studies, paracrystalline or "parking lot" inclusions

   - Example: oculocraniosomatic syndrome (Kearns-Sayre syndrome, ophthalmoplegia plus)

     ○ Retinitis pigmentosa

     ○ Ophthalmoplegia

     ○ Atrial-ventricular (AV) block

     ○ Cerebellar ataxia

     ○ Deafness

     ○ Peripheral neuropathy

     ○ Dwarfism

     ○ Mitochondrial abnormalities in other organs (liver, skin, brain)

     ○ Brain with calcification

   B. Glycogenoses

   - Abnormalities of glycogen metabolism

   - The most common ones to affect skeletal muscle are type II (acid maltase deficiency) and type V (myophosphorylase deficiency, McArdle's disease).

   - Less commonly, other types may affect muscle, including type III (amylo 1,6-glucosidase deficiency, debrancher enzyme), type IV (branching enzyme) and type VII. (phosphofructokinase deficiency)

   - Type II glycogenosis (Pompe's disease)

     ○ Acid maltase deficiency

     ○ Chromosome 17q autosomal recessive condition

     ○ Neonatal form with hypotonia and cardiomegaly, rapidly fatal

     ○ Childhood and adult form with limb–girdle weakness and cardiac disease

     ○ Elevated CPK in all forms

     ○ Type I fibers with vacuoles

     ○ Vacuoles PAS and acid phosphatase (acid maltase is a lysosomal enzyme) positive

     ○ Glycogen accumulation on electron microscopy

   - Type V glycogenosis (McArdle's disease)

     ○ Myophosphorylase deficiency

     ○ Autosomal recessive condition, chromosome 11q

     ○ Males > females

     ○ Muscle cramps and stiffness on exertion

     ○ Abnormal ischemic exercise test—do

not get the expected elevation of blood lactate levels following exercise

- ○ Vacuolar myopathy—typically subsarcolemmal blebs
- ○ Vacuolar PAS positive, acid phosphatase negative

C. Lipid storage myopathies

- Resulting from deficiencies in the carnitine transport system or deficiencies in the mitochondrial dehydrogenase enzyme system
- Related to deficiencies of carnitine, acyl-CoA dehydrogenase, or carnitine palmitoyltransferase (CPT)
- Carnitine deficiency may be either myopathic (limited to muscle) or systemic
- Myopathic carnitine deficiency presents with generalized weakness, usually starting in childhood
- CPT deficiency often presents with myoglobinuria (rhabdomyolysis following exercise)
- Histologically marked by an accumulation of lipid within predominantly type I myocytes (highlighted with oil-red-O or Sudan black stain)

D. Myoadenylate deaminase deficiency

- Intolerance to exercise with cramps, stiffness, or pain
- Autosomal recessive condition
- CPK levels high with exertion
- Type II fibers normally contain more of the enzyme than type I fibers
- Can stain for myoadenylate deaminase to demonstrate deficiency

E. Malignant hyperthermia

- Rapid and sustained rise in temperature during general anesthesia
- Generalized muscle rigidity, tachycardia, cyanosis
- Extensive myonecrosis with subsequent renal failure may develop
- Autosomal dominant condition
- Caffeine or anesthetic stimulation test on muscle strips in vitro
- Muscle pathology nonspecific

F. Channelopathies

- Ion channel myopathies

- Most are autosomal dominant, males > females
- Myotonia, relapsing episodes of hypotonic paralysis following exercise, exposure to cold or high-carbohydrate meal
- Variants recognized associated with varied serum potassium levels (normokalemic, hyperkalemic, or hypokalemic periodic paralysis)
- Myotonia congenita form linked to the chloride channel (chromosome 7)
- Hyperkalemic forms and paramyotonia congenita form (childhood disorder marked by myotonia and hypotonia that increases with continued exercise, especially in the cold) linked to the sodium channel (chromosome 17)
- PAS-positive vacuoles resulting from dilatation of the sarcoplasmic reticulum
- Tubular aggregates, highlighted by NADH stain

VII. Toxic Myopathies

A. Rhabdomyolysis

- Necrosis (degeneration)
- Regeneration
- Scant inflammation
- Rarely calcification
- Seen with drugs, metabolic myopathy, viral myositis, malignant hyperthermia, potassium deficiency, trauma/ischemia, idiopathic
- Caused by drugs and toxic agents, include alcohol, heroin, carbon monoxide, barbiturates, amphetamines, methadone, amphotericin B

B. Subacute necrotizing myopathy—alcohol, AZT, clofibrate

- Ethanol ingestion
- May also cause rhabdomyolysis
- Acute muscle pain that may be generalized or localized

C. Inflammatory—cimetidine, procainamide, D-penicillamine

D. Hypokalemic—diuretics, laxatives, licorice

E. Type IIb fiber atrophy—steroids

F. Vacuolar chloroquine myopathy

- Proximal muscle weakness

- Autophagic membrane bound vacuoles containing membranous debris
- Curvilinear bodies
- Vacuoles more common in type I fibers
- Variable degrees of myocyte necrosis

G. Hyperthyroid myopathy

- Thyrotoxic myopathy—proximal muscle weakness, biopsies often normal
- Hypokalemic periodic paralysis rarely develops with vacuoles
- Associated with myasthenia gravis and exophthalmic ophthalmoplegia

VIII. Muscular Dystrophies

A. Traditionally classified by pattern of inheritance

- X-linked recessive
  - Duchenne
  - Becker
  - Emery-Dreifuss
- Autosomal dominant
  - Facio-scapulo-humeral
  - Myotonic
  - Oculopharyngeal
  - Distal dystrophic myopathy
- Autosomal recessive
  - Limb–girdle (some autosomal dominant)
  - Congenital

B. Many of them are being reclassified based on underlying defects

C. Duchenne dystrophy/Becker dystrophy

- Males
- Rarely spontaneous mutation (about one-third of cases)
- Early-onset pelvic limb–girdle (proximal), wheelchair dependence by age 10–12 yr in Duchenne dystrophy
- Pseudohypertrophic calves—related to increased fat and connective tissue
- CPK increased
- Cardiac involvement (heart failure or arrhythmias)
- Subset of patients have structural abnormalities in the CNS with mental retardation

- Death—early twenties in Duchenne dystrophy
- Becker dystrophy less severe with later age of onset and slower rate of progression with normal life expectancy
- Dystrophin absent in Duchenne dystrophy; decreased or abnormal dystrophin with Becker dystrophy
- Dystrophin gene (chromosome Xq) abnormalites may be result of deletions, point mutations, or frameshift changes
- Dystrophin—a 427 KD protein associated with the sarcolemmal membrane and localized to I and M bands
- Histopathology overlapping between Duchenne and Becker dystrophy
  - Variable muscle fiber size—atrophy and hypertrophy with central nuclei
  - Large ballooned fiber and hypercontracted fibers
  - Nests of regeneration
  - Muscle fiber degeneration
  - Endomysial fibrosis
  - Type I predominance

D. Emery-Dreyfuss dystrophy

- Onset in childhood
- Difficulty in walking, rigidity of neck or spine, elbow deformity
- Slowly progressive
- Cardiac involvement common
- Histopathology marked by myopathic changes such as variation in fiber size, increased central nuclei, degenerating fibers, fibrosis
- Absent emerin by immunohistochemistry

E. Facio-scapulo-humeral dystrophy

- Variable age of onset (usually between ages 10 and 30 yr)
- Weakness of muscles of face, neck, and shoulder girdle
- A subgroup related to defect on chromosome 4q35
- Histopathology characterized by fiber size variation, chronic inflammation, moth-eaten and lobulated fibers

F. Myotonic dystrophy

- Most patients young and middle-aged, most common of adult-onset dystrophies
- Facial, distal amyotrophy of limbs, myotonic (sustained involuntary contractions of muscles) syndrome
- Systemic involvement: frontoparietal balding, cataracts, cardiac disease, hypoplasia of genital organs
- An inherited neonatal form exists
- Gene located on chromosome 19q13 encodes myotonin protein kinase
- Trinucleotide (CTG) repeat disorder
- Histopathology
  - Type I atrophy and type II hypertrophy
  - Chains of nuclei with increased internal nuclei
  - Acid phosphatase hyperactivity
  - Variable fibrosis, degeneration, regeneration
  - Ring fibers common—rim of fiber contains myofibrils that are oriented circumferentially around the longitudinally oriented fibrils in the rest of the fiber

G. Oculopharyngeal dystrophy

- Onset in mid-adult life
- Ptosis and extraocular muscle weakness
- Difficulty swallowing
- Gene defect on chromosome 14q
- Histopathology characterized by vacuoles with tubulofilamentous structures by electron microscopy, variability in fiber size, increased central nuclei

H. Limb–girdle dystrophy

- Wide variety of subtypes recognized as related to different gene defects (caveolin 3, calpain 3, sarcoglycan)
- Onset of different subtypes at different ages
- Weakness of pelvi-femoral muscles and shoulder–girdle muscles
- Pathology marked by fiber splitting, increased central nuclei, variability in fiber size, degenerating fibers, fibrosis, regenerating fibers, moth-eaten fibers, whorled fibers, and ring fibers

I. Congenital muscular dystrophy

- Neonatal hypotonia, respiratory insufficiency, delayed motor milestones, contractures
- A subgroup is merosin negative (related to mutation in the merosin laminin α II gene)
- Pathology marked by variability in fiber size, fibrosis, degenerating and regenerating myofibrers, increased central nuclei

11 Peripheral Nerve

I. General Background

A. Incidence of peripheral neuropathy-40/100,000

B. Clinical patterns include polyneuropathy, mononeuropathy, mononeuropathy multiplex, and plexopathy

C. Etiologies quite variable

- Acquired toxic or metabolic (50%), include such entities as diabetes, alcoholism, vitamin B_{12} deficiency, drug toxicities
- Inflammatory/infectious (10–20%), includes such entities as Guillian-Barre syndrome, chronic inflammatory demyelinating polyradiculopathy, vasculitis, leprosy
- Neoplastic or paraneoplastic (5–10%)
- Genetic/inherited abnormalities (10–20%), includes the hereditary motor and sensory neuropathies
- Unknown (10–20%)

D. Evaluation of the patient with suspected peripheral nerve disease—history (onset, course, other diseases, medications, family history, exposures), physical examination, electrodiagnostic testing with EMG/nerve conduction studies, therapeutic trial, biopsy

E. Procedures involved in handling of the biopsy specimen

- Fixation in formalin (routine light microscopy) and glutaraldehyde (electron microscopy)
- Teased nerve preparation
- Frozen tissue

F. Artifacts associated with biopsy specimen processing

- Stretch trauma—causes myelin splitting

- Crush trauma—causes axonal swelling, gaps in myelin
- Fixation artifacts—formalin fixation may cause "neurokeratin" or herringbone appearance of myelinated fibers, fixation in a hyperosmolar solution may cause shrinkage and loss of circular profile

II. Major Pathologic Processes

A. Axonal (Wallerian) degeneration

- Result of primary destruction of the axon with secondary degeneration of myelin
- Damage to axon may be focal (trauma, ischemia) or more generalized because of abnormalities affecting the neuron cell body (neuronopathy) or axon (axonopathy)
- Wallerian degeneration occurs as result of focal lesion—traumatic transection of nerve
- Distal to site of transection—acute nerve ischemia with inflammation (macrophages to clean up myelin debris)
- Axons undergo alterations of the cytoskeleton and organelles, watery axoplasm
- Myelin undergoes fragmentation forming myelin ovoids with paranodal retraction
- With axonal regeneration, may see a proliferation of Schwann cells within pre-existing basal lamina—bands of Bungner
- A regenerative cluster a result of the growth of one or more growth cones into a band of Bungner
- Eventually, remyelination occurs—new myelin thinner caliber, shortened internodal distances
- Regenerative process slow, limited by the

slowest component of axonal transport (2 mm/d)

B. Distal axonopathy

- "Dying back" axonopathy
- Entire neuron diseased
- Initial changes seen in portion farthest away from the cell body
- Marked by axonal swelling, filamentous inclusions, axonal atrophy, organelle alterations, and Schwann cell networks

C. Demyelination (segmental)

- Primary demyelination related to Schwann cell dysfunction (e.g. diphtheritic neuropathy) or myelin sheath damage
- Degenerating myelin engulfed by Schwann cells and macrophages
- Injured Schwann cells may be replaced by cells in the endoneurium
- Axons surrounded by degenerating myelin or denuded myelin
- Denuded axon provides stimulation for remyelination
- Newly formed myelin of thinner caliber
- Shortened internodal distances with remyelination
- With repeated episodes of demyelination and remyelination, a layering of Schwann cell processes (concentric layers of Schwann cell cytoplasm and basement membrane) around a thinly myelinated axon forms onion bulb
- With chronicity, some degree of axonal injury may occur
- May get secondary demyelination related to axonal injury
- Rare defects of hypomyelination (myelin sheaths thin in all fibers [e.g., hereditary motor and sensory neuropathy type III]) and hypermyelination (abnormal numbers of myelin lamellae often related to folding and reversal of the myelin spiral)

III. Neuropathy Types

A. Traumatic

- May be caused by lacerations (cutting injury), avulsions (pulling apart), or traction
- Regeneration of the transected nerve may be slow, problems related to the discontinuity of the proximal and distal portions of the

nerve sheath and the misalignment of fascicles

- Regrowth may result in a disorganized mass of axons—traumatic or amputation neuroma
- Compression neuropathy related to carpal tunnel syndrome (compression of the median nerve at the level of the wrist)
- In entrapment neuropathies, the compressed region narrowed with nerve expansion proximal to and distal to the region, myelinated fiber size decreased and may see evidence of axonal degeneration and/or demyelination
- Other common sites of compression neuropathy the ulnar nerve at the elbow, peroneal nerve at the knee, radial nerve in the upper arm, and interdigital nerve of the foot at intermetatarsal sites (Morton's neuroma)
- Radiation may cause fiber loss and fibrosis

B. Guillain-Barre syndrome

- AKA: acute inflammatory demyelinating polyradiculopathy
- Overall annual incidence of 1–3/100,000 in United States
- Distal limb weakness, rapidly progressing to more proximal weakness (ascending paralysis)
- Majority of cases with antecedent viral illness
- Deep tendon reflexes diminish
- Decreased nerve conduction velocity
- Elevated CSF protein
- Mortality rate 2–5%, most commonly related to respiratory problem or autonomic instability
- Pathology
  - Endoneurial and perivascular chronic inflammation (lymphocytes, plasma cells and macrophages)
  - Segmental demyelination

C. Chronic inflammatory demyelinating polyradiculopathy (CIDP)

- A subacute or chronic course (at least 8 wk)
- Association with HLA-B8
- Typically marked by relapses and remissions
- Most commonly a symmetric, mixed sensorimotor polyneuropathy
- May respond to steroids or plasmapheresis

- Pathology marked by demyelination pattern of injury with some onion bulb formation developing over time

D. Infectious neuropathies

- Leprosy

    ○ Infection by *Mycobacterium leprae*

    ○ Also affects primarily skin and mucous membranes

    ○ Symmetric polyneuropathy especially involving pain fibers

    ○ Lepromatous leprosy marked by Schwann cell invasion by organisms, segmental demyelination and remyelination, and loss of axons

    ○ With chronicity, fibrosis and perineurial thickening occurs

    ○ Tuberculoid leprosy marked by nodular granulomatous inflammation, particularly affecting cutaneous nerves, sparse numbers of organisms

- Diphtheria

    ○ Neuropathy related to the effects of an exotoxin

    ○ Often presents with weakness and paresthesias, loss of proprioception and vibratory sensation

    ○ Earliest changes observed in the sensory ganglia

    ○ Demyelination changes

- Varicella-zoster

    ○ Affected ganglia marked by neuronal destruction and loss

    ○ Prominent chronic inflammation

    ○ May encounter focal necrosis and hemorrhage

    ○ Axonal degeneration

- Lyme disease

    ○ Caused by infection by *Borrelia burgdorferi* spirochete

    ○ Acquired from a tick bite

    ○ Rash (erythema chronicum migrans), carditis, arthritis

    ○ Frequently affects peripheral nerves

    ○ Perivascular chronic inflammation with axonal degeneration

- HIV

    ○ May encounter acute and chronic polyneuropathies

    ○ May resemble Guillian-Barre disease or CIDP

    ○ Most common HIV-related neuropathy: painful symmetrical sensorimotor neuropathy (mixture of axonal degeneration and demyelination)

    ○ May encounter CMV infection

E. Malignancy—associated neuropathies

- Direct infiltration or compression of nerve by tumor (mononeuropathy)

- Paraneoplastic neuropathy

    ○ Most often encountered with bronchial carcinoma (small cell) associated with IgG anti-Hu antibody

    ○ Subacute sensory neuronopathy or sensorimotor neuropathy

    ○ Depletion of ganglion cells in dorsal root ganglion with a proliferation of capsule cells and perivascular chronic inflammation

- Dysproteinemic neuropathy

    ○ Monoclonal gammopathies of undetermined significance

    ○ Most commonly associated with IgM paraproteins, usually with κ light chain

    ○ Males > females

    ○ Chronic distal sensorimotor neuropathy with tremor and ataxia

    ○ Demyelinative neuropathy with hypertrophic changes and widely spaced myelin

    ○ Anti-myelin-associated protein (MAG) antibodies in 50–90% of cases

F. Hereditary motor and sensory neuropathies (HMSN)

- Charcot-Marie-Tooth disease, hypertrophic type (HMSN I)

    ○ Presents in childhood/early adulthood, slowly progressive

    ○ Autosomal dominant

    ○ Peroneal muscular atrophy, pes cavus

    ○ Three subtypes: IA—duplication on chromosome 17p11.2–p12 peripheral myelin protein 22; IB—chromosome 1 myelin protein zero; IC—not known

○ X-linked variety associated with mutation of gap junction protein gene connexin-32

○ Demyelinating neuropathy with prominent onion bulb formation and hypertrophic changes

- HMSN II

○ Neuronal form of Charcot-Marie-Tooth disease

○ No nerve enlargement as in HMSN I

○ Presents at a slightly later age than HMSN I

○ Chromosome 1p abnormality

○ Loss of axons

- Dejerine-Sottas disease (HMSN III)

○ Slowly progressive, autosomal recessive

○ Presents in early childhood with delayed developmental milestones

○ Trunk and limb muscle involved

○ Nerve enlargement

○ Demyelination with onion bulb formation, some axonal loss

G. Other hereditary neuropathies

- Hereditary sensory and autonomic neuropathies

○ Type I—autosomal dominant, axonal degeneration, sensory neuropathy presenting in adults

○ Type II—autosomal recessive, sensory neuropathy presenting in infancy, axonal degeneration

○ Type III—Riley-Day syndrome, autosomal recessive chromosome 9q, autonomic neuropathy of infancy, axonal degeneration of unmyelinated axons, atrophy and loss of sensory and autonomic ganglia

- Adrenoleukodystrophy

○ X-linked

○ Mixed motor and sensory neuropathy

○ Adrenal insufficiency

○ Spastic paraplegia

○ Axonal degeneration (both myelinated and unmyelinated axons)

○ Segmental demyelination with onion bulbs

○ Linear inclusions in Schwann cells

- Metachromatic leukodystrophy

○ Reduction in myelinated fiber number

○ Segmental demyelination and remyelination

○ Perinuclear granules in Schwann cells, which stain metachromatically—membrane bound, lamellated inclusions (prism stacks, "tuff stone bodies," and zebra bodies)

- Globoid cell leukodystrophy

○ Moderate reduction in myelinated axons

○ Segmental demyelination and remyelination

○ Schwann cells contain straight or curved prism/tubular inclusions

- Refsum's disease

○ Phytanoyl CoA α-hydroxylase abnormality (peroxisomal enzyme)

○ Autosomal recessive

○ Onset before age 20 yr

○ Ataxia, night-blindness, retinitis pigmentosa, ichthyosis

○ Hypertrophic nerves, mixed motor and sensory neuropathy

○ Prominent onion bulb formation

- Porphyria

○ Peripheral nerve involvement with acute intermittent and variegate coproporphyria types

○ Autosomal dominant

○ Acute episodes of neurologic dysfunction, psychiatric abnormalities, abdominal pain, seizures, autonomic dysfunction, proximal weakness

○ Distal axonopathy of "dying back" type

H. Nutritional deficiency/toxic neuropathies

- Beriberi (thiamine deficiency)

○ Distal, symmetrical sensorimotor neuropathy

○ Axonal loss and degeneration distally

- ○ Secondary segmental demyelination more proximally
- ○ Alcoholic neuropathy has a similar pathologic appearance
- Vitamin B$_{12}$ deficiency
  - ○ Symmetrical sensory polyneuropathy
  - ○ May not necessarily be associated with subacute combined degeneration of the cord
  - ○ Axonal degeneration
- Vitamin E deficiency
  - ○ Spinocerebellar degeneration and sensory neuropathy
  - ○ Related to chronic intestinal fat malabsorption
  - ○ Loss of myelinated axons
- Toxic neuropathies
  - ○ A wide spectrum of toxic neuropathies
  - ○ Diagnoses depend on excluding other causes of neuropathy

I. Miscellaneous neuropathies
- Diabetic neuropathy
  - ○ Wide variety of diseases may be encountered: distal symmetric or sensorimotor neuropathy, autonomic neuropathy (20–40% of diabetics), focal/multifocal asymmetric neuropathy
  - ○ Decreased sensation in distal extremities
  - ○ Prevalence of peripheral neuropathy related to duration of disease
  - ○ Almost all patients with conduction abnormalities
  - ○ Predominant pathology: axonal neuropa-

thy accompanied by some segmental demyelination
  - ○ Arteriolar thickening
- Uremic neuropathy
  - ○ Distal, symmetric neuropathy
  - ○ May be asymptomatic or associated with muscle cramps, dysesthesias, and decreased deep tendon reflexes
  - ○ Axonal degeneration
  - ○ Regeneration and some recovery after dialysis
- Amyloid neuropathy
  - ○ May encounter with myeloma, Waldenström's macroglobulinemia
  - ○ Hereditary syndromes exist—most commonly related to mutations in transthyretin (prealbumin) gene
  - ○ Hereditary forms most commonly autosomal dominant, often marked by sensory and autonomic dysfunction
  - ○ Amyloid deposits primarily in vessel walls with axonal degeneration
  - ○ Neuropathy usually not associated with secondary amyloidosis
- Vasculitic neuropathy
  - ○ Axonal degeneration
  - ○ May be related to a variety of different vasculitic processes: polyarteritis nodosa (necrotizing), Churg-Strauss, collagen–vascular disease
- Sarcoidosis
  - ○ May be multifocal
  - ○ Perivascular or endoneurial non-necrotizing granulomas
  - ○ Nerve findings nonspecific

12 Figures with Questions

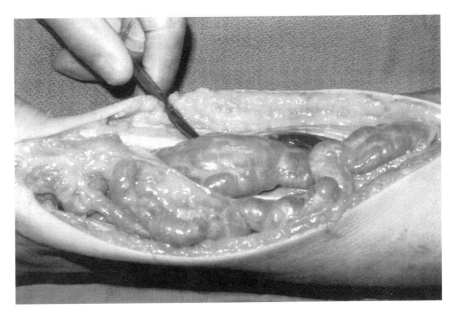

Question 1

1. The lesion shown here is almost exclusively seen
   in the setting of
   A. Neurofibromatosis type I
   B. Neurofibromatosis type II
   C. Tuberous sclerosis
   D. Neurocutaneous melanosis
   E. Li-Fraumeni syndrome

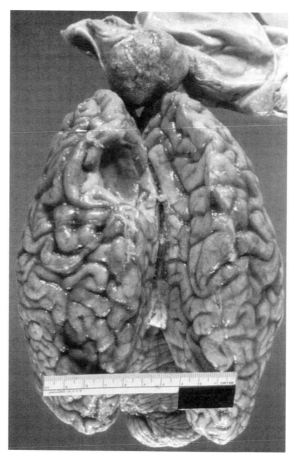

Question 2

2. The most common cytogenetic abnormality associated with this lesion is related to chromosome
   A. 1
   B. 6
   C. 9
   D. 17
   E. 22

3. The most likely diagnosis is
   A. Metastatic carcinoma
   B. Lymphoma
   C. Glioblastoma multiforme
   D. Meningioma
   E. Medulloblastoma

4. This lesion presented as a lateral ventricular mass in an 18-yr-old male with seizures and adenoma sebaceum. The lesion represents a
   A. Cortical tuber
   B. Subependymal giant-cell astrocytoma
   C. Hemangioma
   D. Neurofibroma
   E. Hemangioblastoma

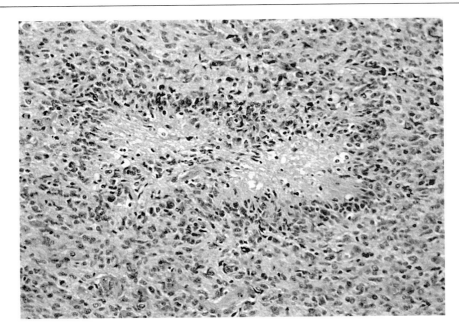

Question 3

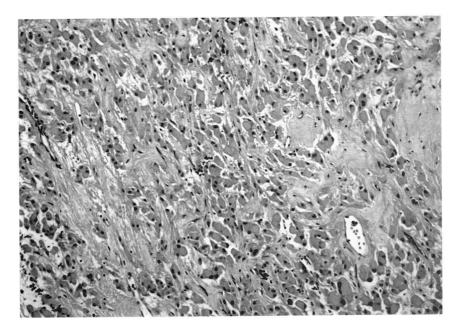

Question 4

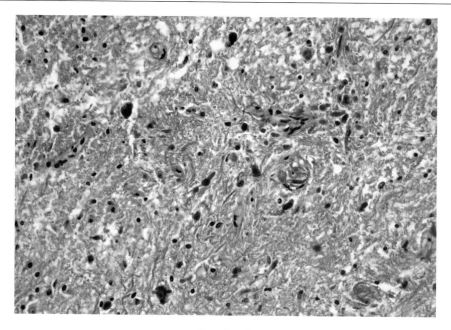

Question 5

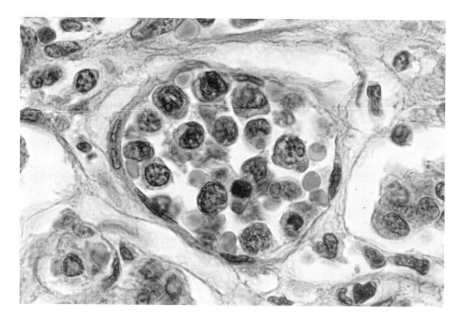

Question 6

5. These brightly eosinophilic staining, irregularly shaped structures in a pilocytic astrocytoma are referred to as

   A. Rosenthal fibers

   B. Granular bodies

   C. Marinesco bodies

   D. Tangles

   E. None of the above

6. The cells in the intravascular lesion stain positively with CD20. The diagnosis

   A. Metastatic carcinoma

   B. Metastatic pituitary adenoma

   C. Vasculitis

   D. Lymphoma

   E. Histiocytosis X

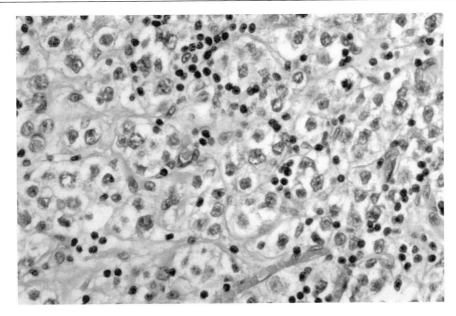

Question 7

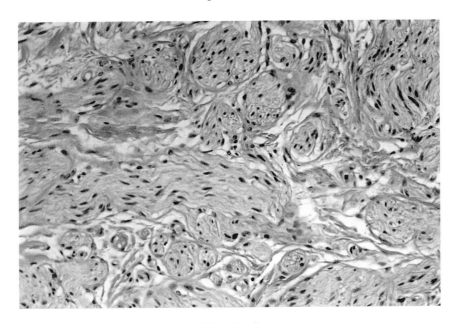

Question 8

7. This lesion represents a pineal gland mass in a 17-yr-old male.

   A. Lymphoma

   B. Pineocytoma

   C. Germinoma

   D. Pineoblastoma

   E. Epithelioid glioma

8. This right arm lesion in an area of previous trauma represents a

   A. Neurofibroma

   B. Schwannoma

   C. Morton's neuroma

   D. Traumatic neuroma

   E. Paraganglioma

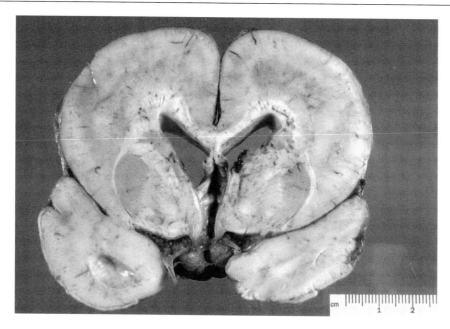

Question 9

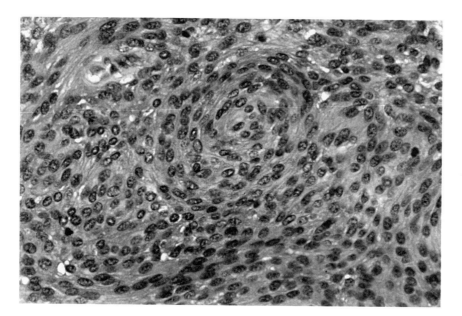

Question 10

9. The malformation illustrated is best denoted as
   A. Lissencephaly
   B. Polymicrogyria
   C. Schizencephaly
   D. Periventricular leukomalacia
   E. Hydranencephaly

10. This lesion is best classified as a(n)
   A. Astrocytoma
   B. Ependymoma
   C. Meningioma
   D. Metastatic carcinoma
   E. Schwannoma

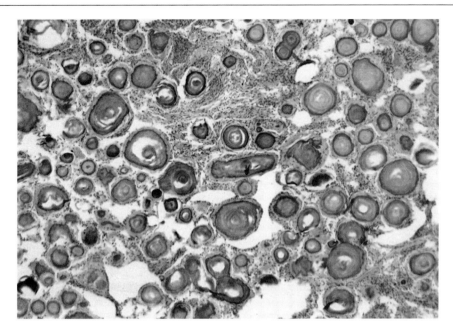

Question 11

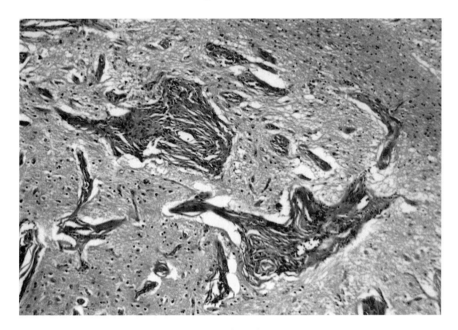

Question 12

11. The numerous round to oval calcified structures in this tumor are termed
    A. Calcified parasite eggs
    B. Marinesco bodies
    C. Hyaline bodies
    D. Psammoma bodies
    E. Corpora amylacea

12. Collars of perivascular meningothelial cells mark this lesion, which is most commonly seen associated with
    A. Neurofibromatosis type I
    B. Neurofibromatosis type II
    C. Tuberous sclerosis
    D. von Hippel-Lindau disease
    E. Sturge-Weber disease

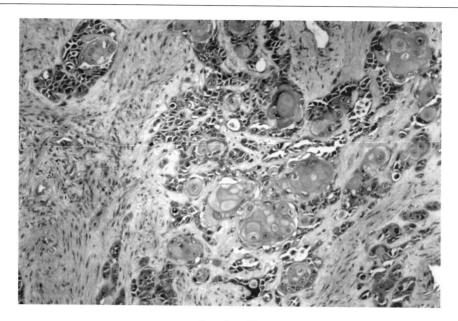

Question 13

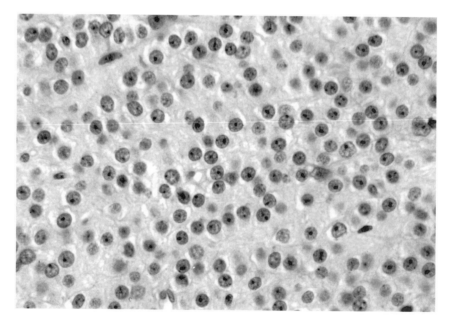

Question 14

13. This lesion is extending into the dura from an adjacent sinus. The diagnosis is

    A. Mucor infection

    B. Aspergillus infection

    C. Squamous cell carcinoma

    D. Meningioma

    E. Adenocarcinoma

14. This lateral ventricular mass in a 32-yr-old male stains positively with synaptophysin and negatively with GFAP. The diagnosis is

    A. Oligodendroglioma

    B. Clear cell ependymoma

    C. Neurocytoma

    D. Subependymal giant-cell astrocytoma

    E. Subependymoma

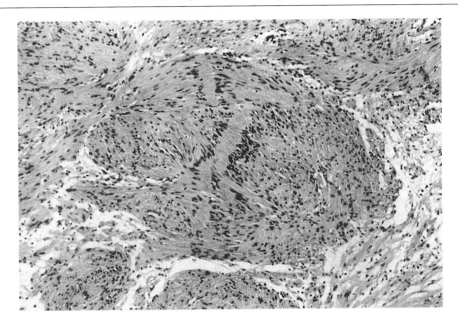

Question 15

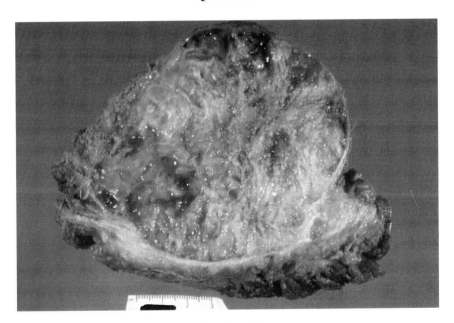

Question 16

15. The diagnosis is

    A. Anaplastic astrocytoma

    B. Schwannoma

    C. Ependymoma

    D. Neurofibroma

    E. Leiomyoma

16. This bone-based, sacrococcygeal mass microscopically consists of vacuolated epithelioid cells arranged against a mucoid matrix. The most likely diagnosis is

    A. Chordoma

    B. Paraganglioma

    C. Syncytial meningioma

    D. Myxopapillary ependymoma

    E. Teratoma

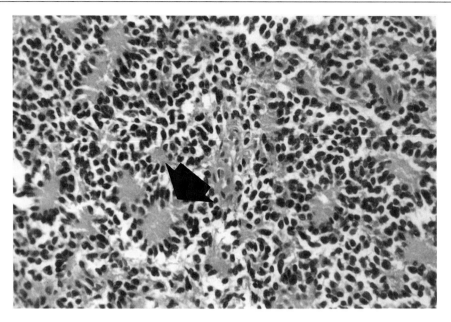

Question 17

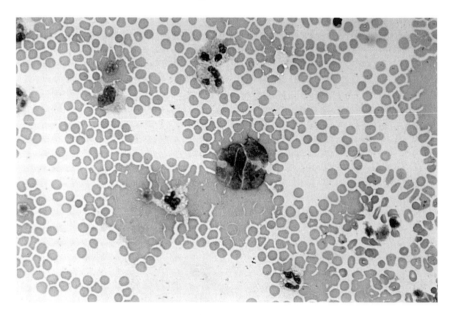

Question 18

17. The structure marked by an arrow in this cerebellar mass in a 6-yr-old is a

   A. Fleurette

   B. Homer Wright rosette

   C. Flexner Wintersteiner rosette

   D. Perivascular pseudorosette

   E. None of the above

18. Cerebrospinal fluid cytology shows atypical cells from a 4-yr-old male's cerebellar mass (synaptophysin positive). The diagnosis is

   A. Ependymoma

   B. Pilocytic astrocytoma

   C. Medulloblastoma

   D. Choroid plexus papilloma

   E. Neurocytoma

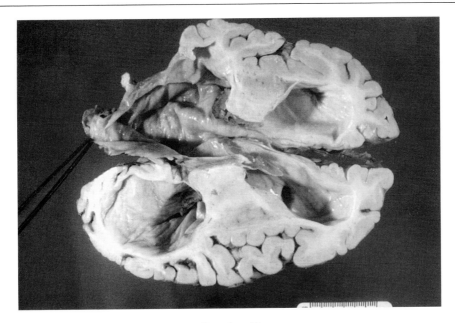

Question 19

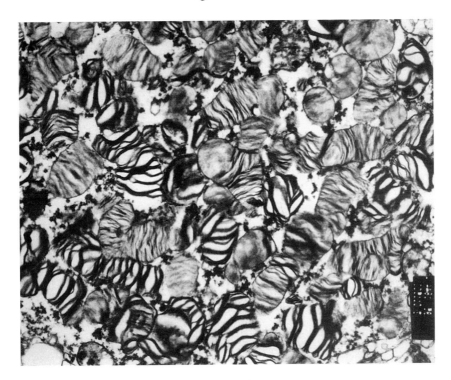

Question 20

19. The lesion illustrated in this 4-yr-old with cerebral palsy is most likely the result of a

   A. Storage disease

   B. Vascular insult

   C. Tumor

   D. Hemorrhage

   E. Inherited syndrome

20. The ultrastructural finding here is from a Tay-Sachs disease patient and is known as

   A. Whorled membrane bodies

   B. Granular bodies

   C. Fingerprint bodies

   D. Curvilinear bodies

   E. Zebra bodies

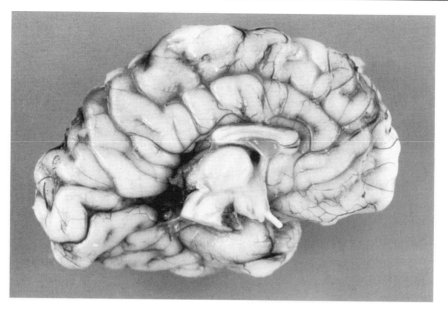

Question 21

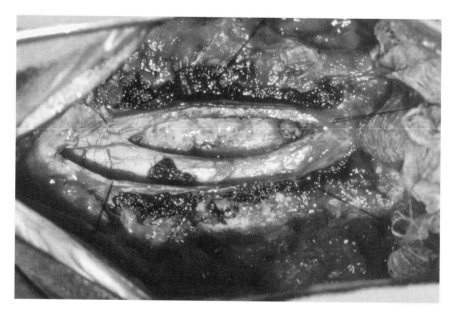

Question 22

21. The defect seen here is best classified as
    A. Agenesis of the corpus callosum
    B. Partial agenesis of the corpus callosum
    C. Polymicrogyria
    D. Dandy-Walker syndrome
    E. Schizencephaly

22. The most likely diagnosis for this well-circumscribed intramedullary spinal cord mass is
    A. Schwannoma
    B. Meningioma
    C. Astrocytoma
    D. Ependymoma
    E. Oligodendroglioma

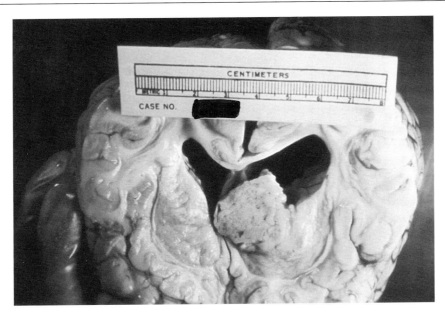

Question 23

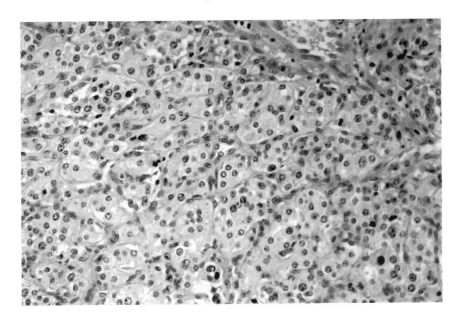

Question 24

23. The most likely diagnosis in this 8-yr-old female with tuberous sclerosis is

    A. Cortical tuber

    B. Cortical dysplasia

    C. Subependymal giant-cell astrocytoma

    D. Metastatic germ cell tumor

    E. Angiomyolipoma

24. This intradural, chromogranin-positive mass in the cauda equina region represents a

    A. Paraganglioma

    B. Schwannoma

    C. Myxopapillary ependymoma

    D. Meningioma

    E. Chordoma

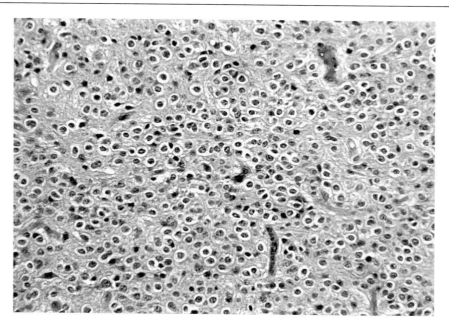

Question 25

25. The most common location for this lesion is

    A. Frontal lobe

    B. Parietal lobe

    C. Occipital lobe

    D. Temporal lobe

    E. Cerebellum

26. The best diagnosis for this lesion is

    A. Herniation

    B. Duret hemorrhage

    C. Chiari malformation

    D. Brain stem glioma

    E. Dandy-Walker syndrome

27. What is the diagnosis?

    A. Metastatic carcinoma

    B. Craniopharyngioma

    C. Pituitary adenoma

    D. Meningioma

    E. Astrocytoma

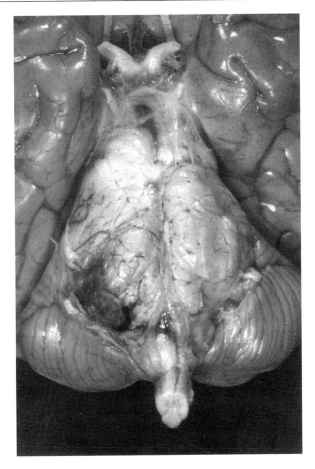

Question 26

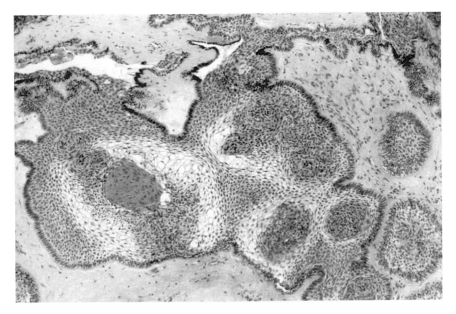

Question 27

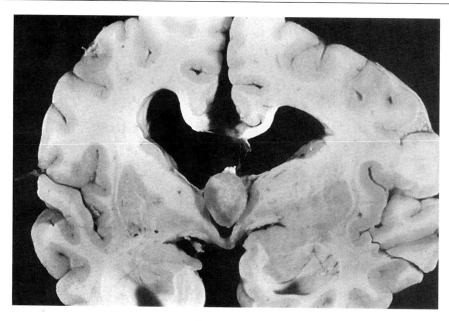

Question 28

28. The most likely diagnosis is
    A. Colloid cyst
    B. Rathke's cleft cyst
    C. Neurenteric cyst
    D. Arachnoid cyst
    E. Endodermal cyst

29. The most likely location for this tumor in a 12-yr-old is
    A. Frontal lobe
    B. 4th ventricle
    C. Cerebellum
    D. Lateral ventricle
    E. Temporal lobe

30. The most likely diagnosis for this tumor that is cytokeratin AE1/3 negative, S-100 protein positive is
    A. Metastatic lung carcinoma
    B. Glioblastoma multiforme
    C. Melanoma
    D. Lymphoma
    E. None of the above

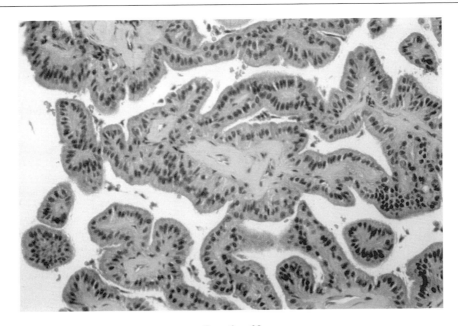

Question 29

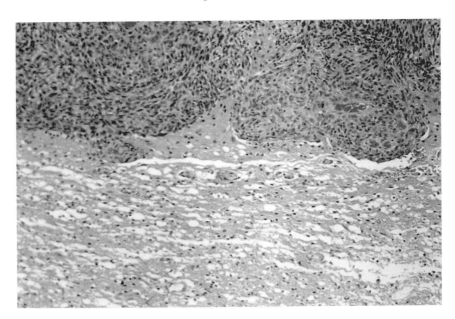

Question 30

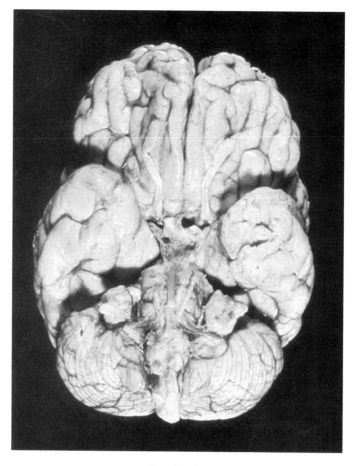

Question 31

31. Which chromosome is affected in this disorder?

    A. 17

    B. 9

    C. 16

    D. 3

    E. 22

32. The most likely hormone secreted by this lesion would be

    A. Prolactin

    B. Growth hormone

    C. ACTH

    D. TSH

    E. FSH

33. The abnormality seen is most likely associated with which of the following?

    A. Neu-Laxova syndrome

    B. Zellweger's syndrome

    C. Walker-Warburg syndrome

    D. Cerebro-ocular dysplasia

    E. Lissencephaly

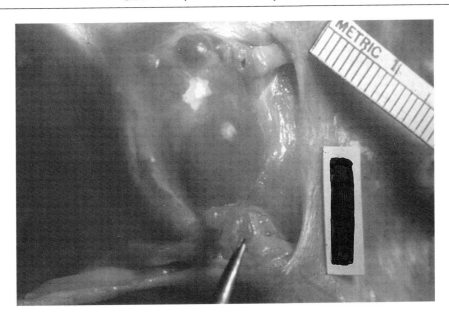

Question 32

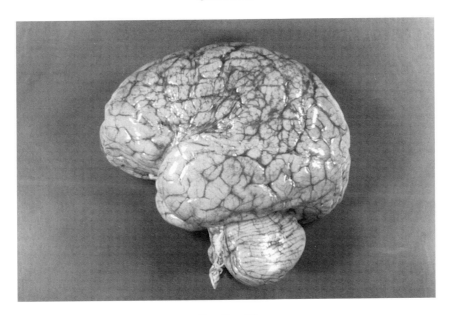

Question 33

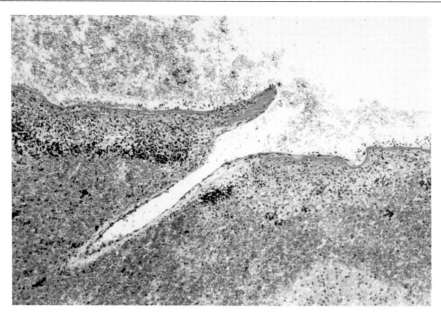

Question 34

34. The hemorrhage seen here in the periventricular region is most likely to occur in a(n)

    A. <32-wk-gestation premature infant

    B. Full-term infant

    C. 1-mo-old infant

    D. 1-yr-old infant

    E. An adult

35. The lesion seen here represents

    A. Multiple sclerosis

    B. Huntington's chorea

    C. Multisystem atrophy

    D. Agenesis of the septum pellucidum

    E. Cavum septi pellucidi

36. The spinal cord tumor seen here ultrastructurally is best classified as

    A. Astrocytoma

    B. Ependymoma

    C. Meningioma

    D. Schwannoma

    E. Paraganglioma

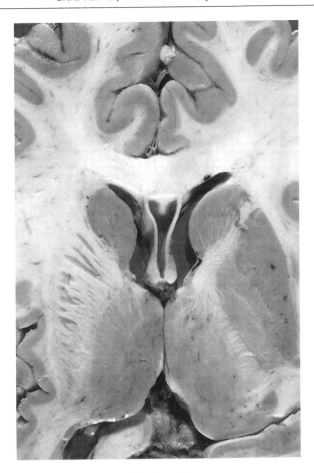

Question 35

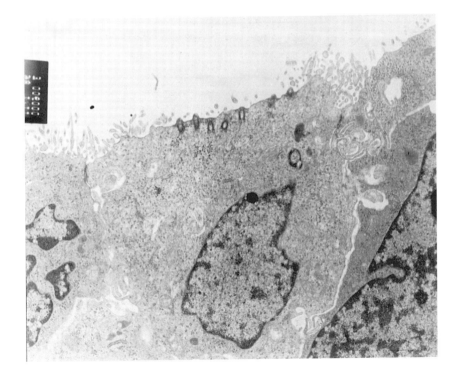

Question 36

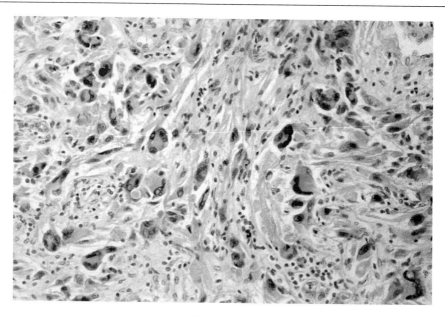

Question 37

37. This temporal lobe tumor arose in a 14-yr-old with a history of chronic epilepsy. The MIB-1 labeling index was <1%. The most likely diagnosis is

    A. Pleomorphic xanthoastrocytoma

    B. Glioblastoma multiforme

    C. Dysembryoplastic neuroepithelial tumor

    D. Pilocytic astrocytoma

    E. Ependymoma

38. A reticulin stain highlights spindled cell areas of this tumor. Nonspindled areas stain with GFAP. The tumor demonstrates focal vascular proliferation and necrosis. The best diagnosis is

    A. Malignant oligodendroglioma

    B. Malignant ependymoma

    C. Gliosarcoma

    D. Metastatic carcinoma

    E. Lymphoma

39. The changes seen here are most characteristic of

    A. Dandy-Walker syndrome

    B. Chiari malformation

    C. Brain stem glioma

    D. Dentate dysplasia

    E. Down's syndrome

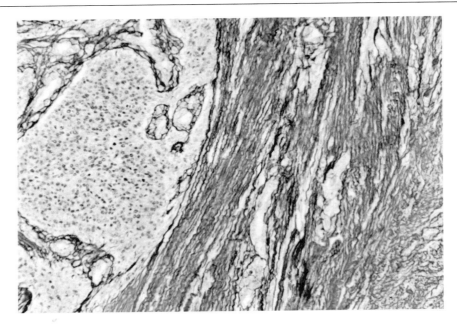

Question 38

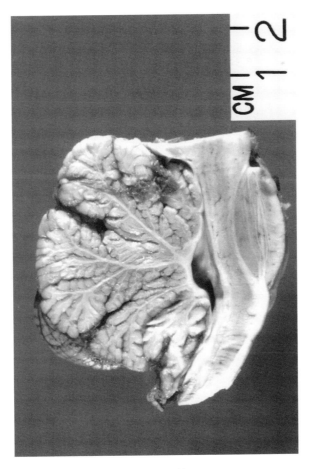

Question 39

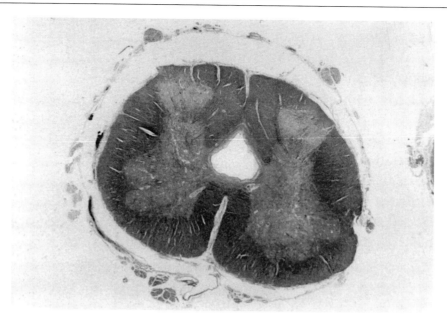

Question 40

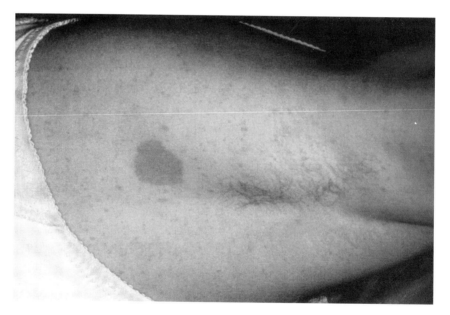

Question 41

40. The ependymal-lined cavity in this section of spinal cord is best termed

A. Syrinx

B. Syringobulbia

C. Aqueductal malformation

D. Hydromyelia

E. Diplomyelia

41. This patient is likely to have all the following except

A. Lisch nodules

B. Pheochromocytoma

C. Sphenoid dysplasia

D. Neurofibroma

E. Subependymal giant cell astrocytoma

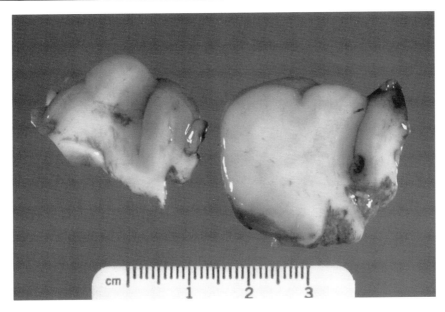

Question 42

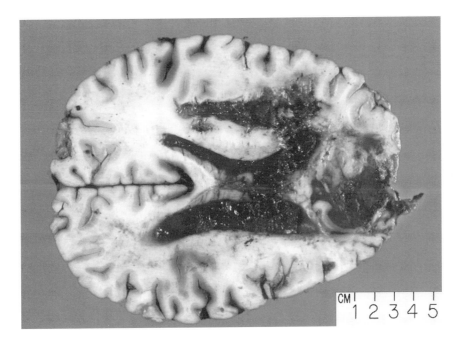

Question 43

42. The gross appearance is most typical for a(n)

A. Infiltrating low-grade glioma

B. Encephalitis

C. Demyelinating disease

D. Pick's disease

E. Infarct

43. Which tumor is most likely to present like this?

A. Low-grade astrocytoma

B. Low-grade oligodendroglioma

C. Ependymoma

D. Ganglioglioma

E. Pilocytic astrocytoma

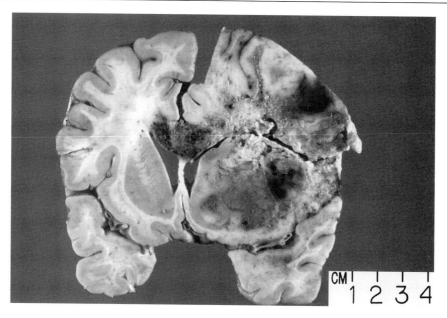

Question 44

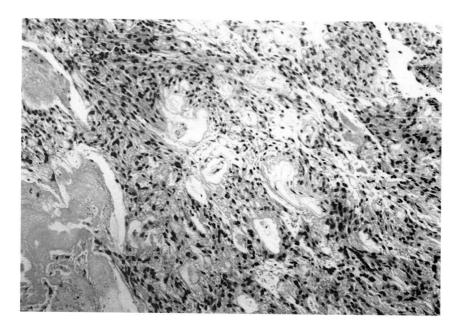

Question 45

44. The best diagnosis for this lesion in a 77-yr-old male is

    A. Remote infarct

    B. Demyelinating disease

    C. Glioblastoma multiforme

    D. Hemorrhage

    E. Fat emboli

45. This GFAP-positive filum terminale mass represents a(n)

    A. Subependymoma

    B. Ependymoma

    C. Myxopapillary ependymoma

    D. Astrocytoma

    E. Schwannoma

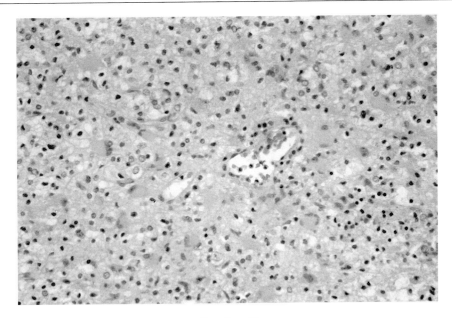

Question 46

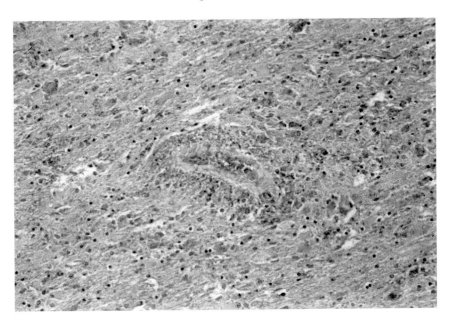

Question 47

46. This 32-yr-old female has multiple white matter lesions that look like this. Her diagnosis is

A. Infarct

B. Multiple sclerosis

C. Anaplastic astrocytoma

D. Vasculitis

E. Storage disease

47. The infant has megalencephaly with diffuse white matter abnormalities. The most likely diagnosis is

A. Alexander's disease

B. Adrenoleukodystrophy

C. Krabbe's disease

D. Metachromatic leukodystrophy

E. Cockayne's disease

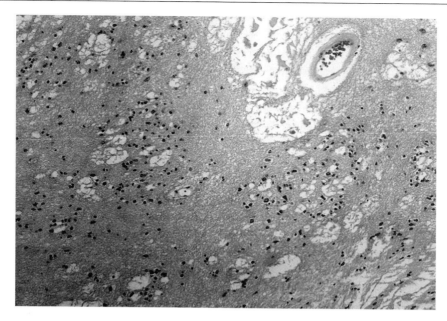

Question 48

48. This mass arose in the floor of the 4th ventricle and was an incidental findings at autopsy. The best diagnosis is

    A. Neurocytoma

    B. Ependymoma

    C. Choroid plexus papilloma

    D. Subependymoma

    E. Meningioma

49. The most likely diagnosis in this 28-yr-old immunocompetent female is

    A. Multiple infarcts

    B. Vasculitis

    C. Astrocytoma

    D. Multiple sclerosis

    E. Progressive multifocal leukoencephalopathy

50. The region denoted by the arrow represents

    A. Dentate

    B. CA4

    C. CA3

    D. Sommer sector

    E. Subiculum

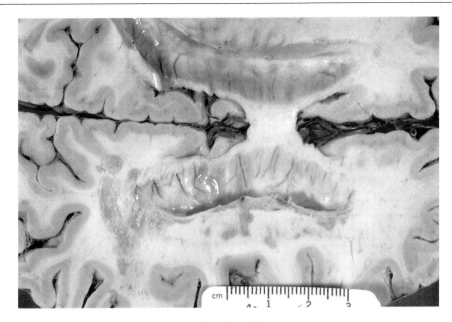

Question 49

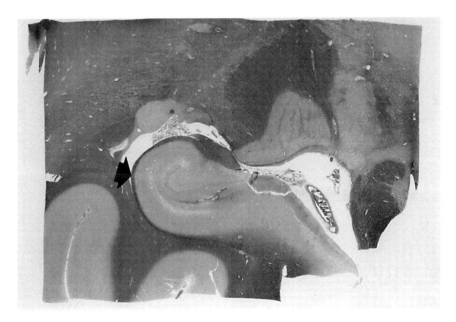

Question 50

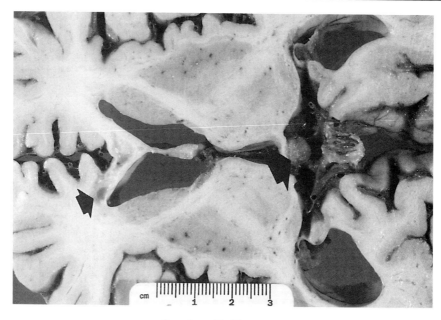

Questions 51, 52, and 53

51. The patient is an 82-yr-old female with dementia. The changes illustrated in this figure are characteristic of

    A. Malformation

    B. Atrophy

    C. Tumor

    D. Demyelinating disease

    E. Hemorrhage

52. (See Figure 51) The lesion denoted by the smaller arrows most likely represents a(n)

    A. Infarct

    B. Malformation

    C. Multiple sclerosis

    D. Low-grade astrocytoma

    E. Microglial nodule

53. (See Figure 51) The lesion denoted by the larger arrow is

    A. Germinoma

    B. Part of a malformation

    C. Colloid cyst

    D. Pineal gland

    E. Pituitary gland

54. The cell denoted by the arrow represents a(n)

    A. Neuron

    B. Oligodendrocyte

    C. Ependymal cell

    D. Endothelial cell

    E. Microglial cell

55. The organism denoted by the smaller arrow represents

    A. CMV

    B. PML

    C. Toxoplasmosis

    D. Amebiasis

    E. Cysticercosis

56. (See Figure 55) The larger arrow denotes an aggregate of cells forming what structure?

    A. Granuloma

    B. Dürcks node

    C. Microglial nodule

    D. Abscess

    E. Sulfur granule

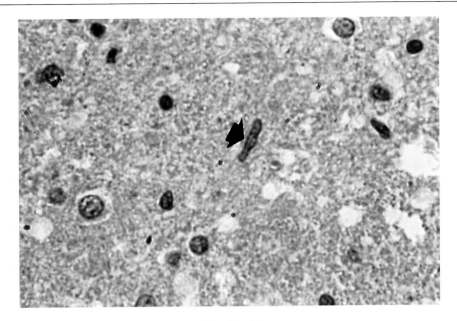

Question 54

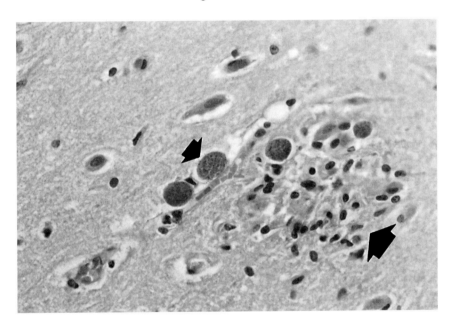

Questions 55 and 56

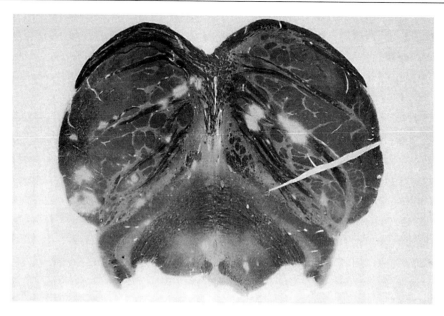

Question 57

57. This patient is a 62-yr-old male with a history of
non-Hodgkin's lymphoma who developed multiple white matter lesions in both the brain and
brain stem. The most likely diagnosis is
    A. SSPE
    B. PML
    C. Multiple sclerosis
    D. CMV
    E. Toxoplasmosis

58. The infectious agent represented in this photomicrograph is
    A. Cryptococcus
    B. Candida
    C. Blastomycosis
    D. CMV
    E. Papova virus

59. (See Figure 58) The process shown represents
    A. Abscess
    B. Ventriculitis
    C. Meningitis
    D. Infarct
    E. Encephalitis

60. The structures seen here represent infection from
    A. Cryptococcus
    B. Candida
    C. Aspergillus
    D. Mucormycosis
    E. Actinomyces

61. (See Figure 60) All of the following organisms
may have hyphae which look like this, except
    A. Rhizopus
    B. Absidia
    C. Mucor
    D. Apophysomyces
    E. Fusarium

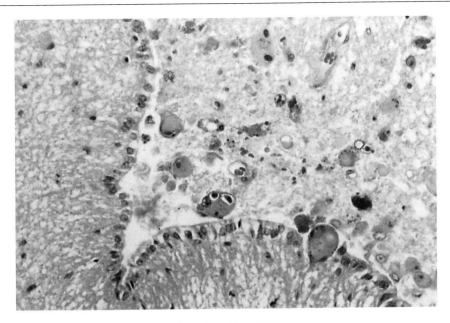

Questions 58 and 59

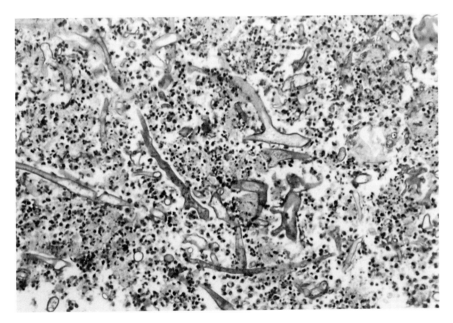

Questions 60 and 61

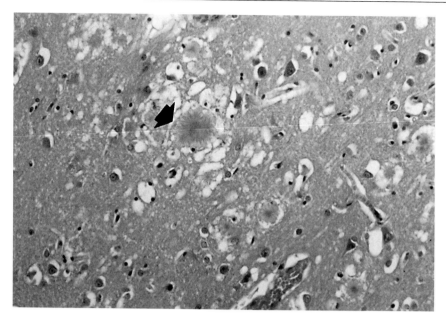

Questions 62 and 63

62. The best diagnosis for this 48-yr-old male with rapidly progressive dementia and myoclonus is
    A. Alzheimer's disease
    B. Pick's disease
    C. Parkinson's disease
    D. Progressive supranuclear palsy
    E. None of the above

63. (See Figure 62) The structure denoted by the arrow represents a(n)
    A. Neurofibrillary tangle
    B. Neuritic plaque
    C. Kuru plaque
    D. Axon torpedo
    E. Granular body

64. The strucuture denoted by the arrow represents
    A. Marinesco body
    B. Hyaline body
    C. Rosenthal fiber
    D. Corpora amylacea
    E. Alzheimer type I astrocyte

65. The structures located in the cytoplasm of the neuron marked by the arrow represent
    A. Pick bodies
    B. Granulovacuolar degeneration
    C. Neurofibrillary tangles
    D. Hirano bodies
    E. Lewy bodies

66. (See Figure 65) The lesion depicted here is most likely to be encountered in the setting of
    A. Alzheimer's disease
    B. Pick's disease
    C. Parkinson's disease
    D. Corticobasal degeneration
    E. Amyotrophic lateral sclerosis

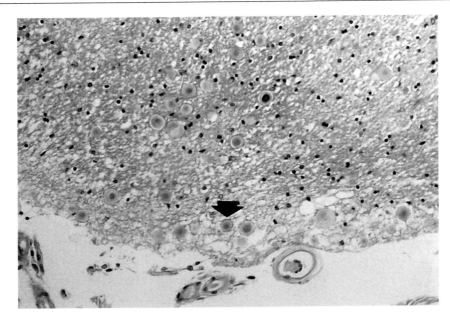

Question 64

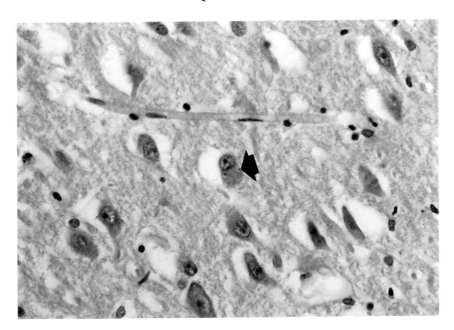

Questions 65 and 66

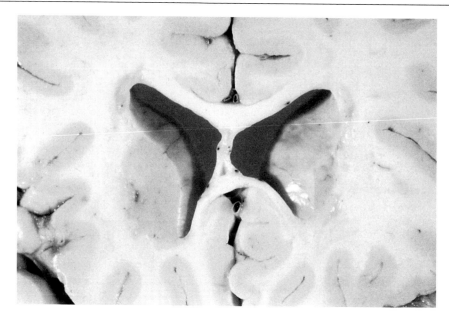

Question 67

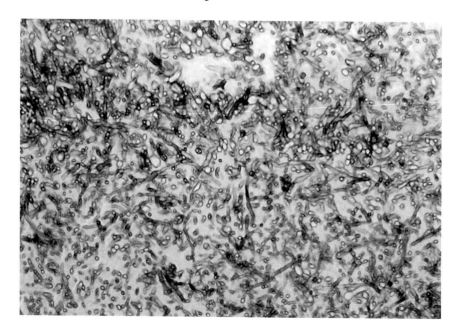

Question 68

67. This 29-yr-old female most likely has
    A. Multiple sclerosis
    B. Glioblastoma multiforme
    C. Cortical dysplasia
    D. Leukodystrophy
    E. Cavum septum pellucidum

68. The organism seen here represents
    A. Candida
    B. Aspergillus
    C. Mucormycosis
    D. Blastomycosis
    E. Cryptococcus

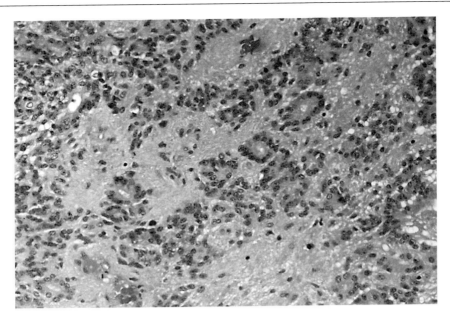

Question 69

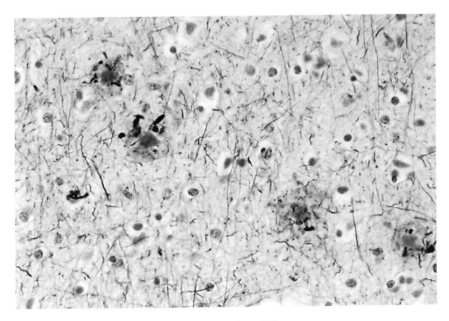

Questions 70 and 71

69. This GFAP-positive intramedullary spinal cord mass represents a(n)

    A. Astrocytoma

    B. Ependymoma

    C. Meningioma

    D. Medulloblastoma

    E. Myxopapillary ependymoma

70. The structures seen here represent

    A. Pick bodies

    B. Granular bodies

    C. Neuritic plaques

    D. Neurofibrillary tangles

    E. Hirano bodies

71. (See Figure 70) The stains most useful to highlight these structures include

    A. Bodian and Congo red

    B. GMS and PAS

    C. GMS and Congo red

    D. Bodian and PAS

    E. Ziehl-Neelson and Congo red

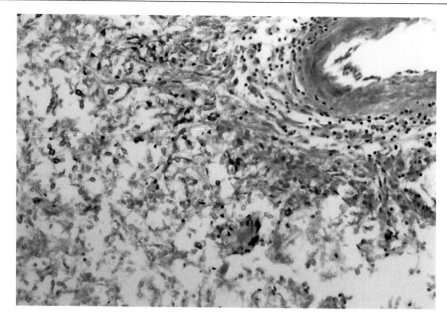

Question 72

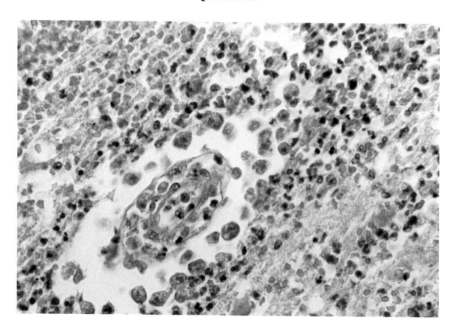

Question 73

72. The mucicarmine-positive organisms seen here represent
    A. Candida
    B. Cryptococcus
    C. Aspergillus
    D. Nocardia
    E. Actinomyces

73. The organism present here represents
    A. Amebiasis
    B. Malaria
    C. Toxoplasmosis
    D. Cysticercosis
    E. Schistosomiasis

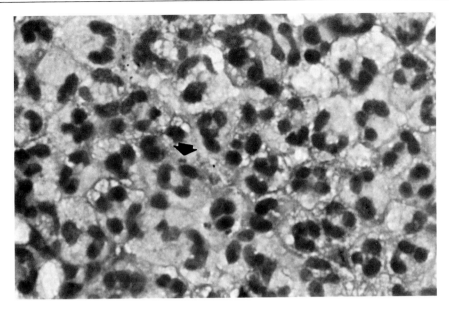

Question 74

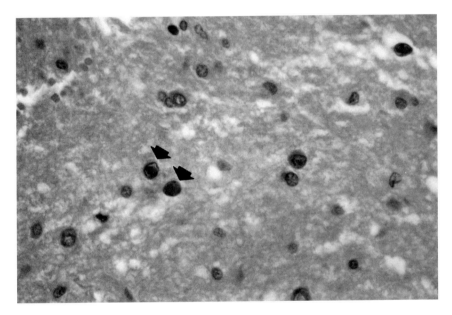

Question 75 and 76

74. The organism denoted by the arrow in this meningitis most likely represents
    A. Meningococcus
    B. *E. coli*
    C. *M. tuberculosis*
    D. Nocardia
    E. Actinomyces

75. The lesions denoted by the arrows represent
    A. Microglial nodules
    B. Cowdry type A inclusions
    C. Cowdry type B inclusions
    D. Cowdry type C inclusions
    E. Cytoplasmic viral inclusions

76. (See Figure 75) The inclusions seen here are caused by the JC virus. Which of the following is a likely finding on the biopsy?
    A. Neutrophilic infiltrate
    B. Alzheimer type I astrocytes
    C. Alzheimer type II astrocytes
    D. Abscess
    E. Microglial nodules

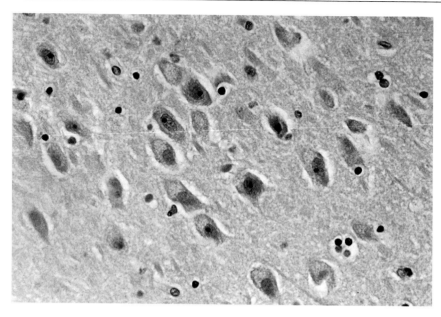

Question 77

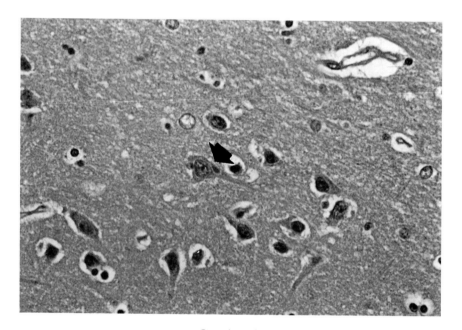

Question 78

77. The cytoplasm of these neurons in this normal
    brain section are filled with

    A. Neuromelanin

    B. Lipofucsin

    C. Hyaline bodies

    D. Marinesco bodies

    E. Hemosiderin

78. The viral inclusion seen in the neuron denoted by
    the arrow represents what infection?

    A. Herpes simplex

    B. Cytomegalovirus

    C. Herpes zoster

    D. SSPE

    E. Rabies

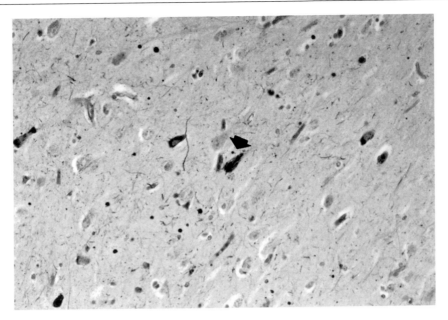

Questions 79 and 80

79. The structure denoted by the arrow on this Bodian-stained section represents

A. Ganulovacuolar degeneration

B. Neuritic plaque

C. Neurofibrillary tangle

D. Hirano body

E. Pick body

80. (See Figure 79) The structure seen here has been described in all of the following conditions except

A. Alzheimer's disease

B. SSPE

C. Parkinson's disease

D. Herpes encephalitis

E. Dementia pugilistica

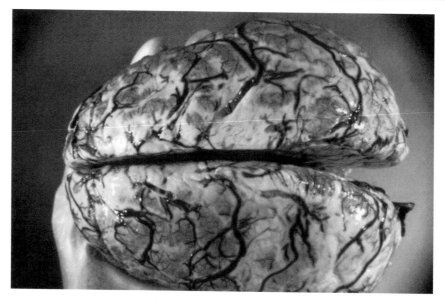

Questions 81, 82, and 83

81. All of the following are abnormalities evident in this photomicrograph except

    A. Vascular congestion

    B. Herniation

    C. Widening of the gyri

    D. Narrowing of the sulci

    E. Meningeal clouding

82. (See Figure 81) All are potential complications of the process seen here except

    A. Ventriculitis

    B. Infarct

    C. Hemorrhage

    D. Secondary glioma development

    E. Hydrocephalus

83. (See Figure 81) The most likely causative organism in a 78-yr-old individual who has not been recently hospitalized would be

    A. *E. coli*

    B. Proteus

    C. Listeria

    D. *S. pneumoniae*

    E. *N. meningitidis*

84. The structure illustrated represents

    A. Choroid plexus

    B. Choroid plexus papilloma

    C. Choroid plexus carcinoma

    D. Papillary meningioma

    E. Papillary ependymoma

85. The cell denoted by the arrow represents a(n)

    A. Astrocyte

    B. Oligodendrocyte

    C. Neuron

    D. Microglial cell

    E. Arachnoidal cap cell

86. (See Figure 85) This cell is most likely to stain positively with which antibody?

    A. GFAP

    B. Synaptophysin

    C. Epithelial membrane antigen

    D. Common leukocyte antigen

    E. HAM 56

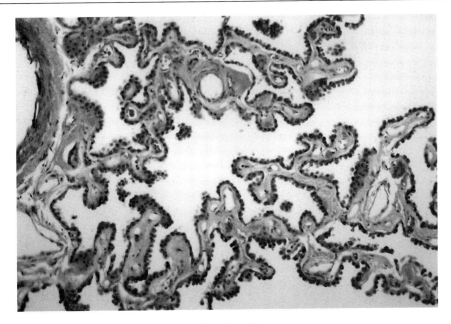

Question 84

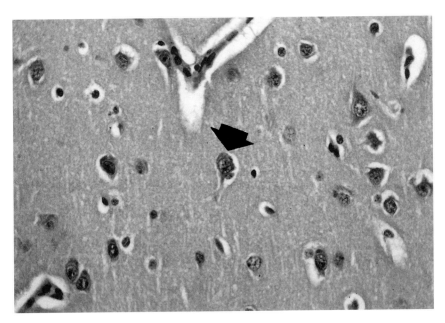

Questions 85 and 86

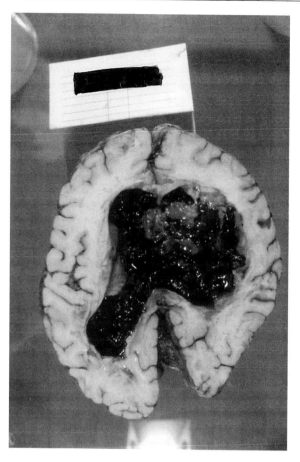

Question 87

87. The most likely cause of hemorrhage in this 58-yr-old male is

    A. Hypertension

    B. Amyloid

    C. Vasculitis

    D. Aneurysm

    E. Oligodendroglioma

88. This leptomeningeal-based lesion is a common CNS finding in

    A. Neurofibromatosis type I

    B. Neurofibromatosis type II

    C. von Hippel-Lindau syndrome

    D. Tuberous sclerosis

    E. Sturge-Weber disease

89. (See Figure 88) The pattern of inheritance associated with this condition is likely to be

    A. X-linked recessive

    B. X-linked dominant

    C. Autosomal dominant

    D. Autosomal recessive

    E. None of the above

90. The illustration most accurately represents a(n)

    A. Tumor

    B. Embolized vascular formation

    C. Artery with vasculitis

    D. Infarct

    E. Aneurysm

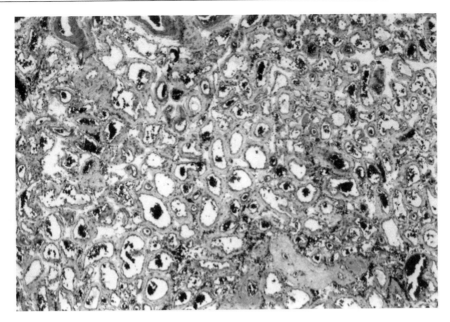

Questions 88 and 89

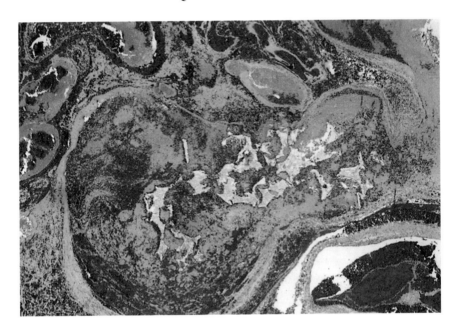

Question 90

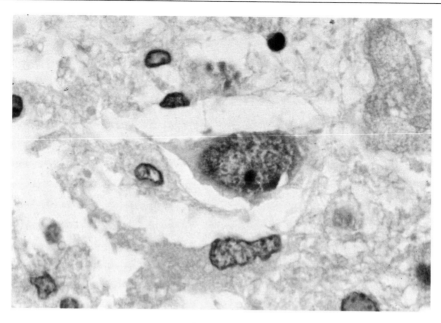

Question 91

91. The large cell seen here in a patient with progressive multifocal leukoencephalopathy represents a(n)

   A. Oligodendrocyte

   B. Neuron

   C. Alzheimer type I astrocyte

   D. Alzheimer type II astrocyte

   E. Cowdry type A inclusion

92. The lesion denoted by the arrows represents a(n)

   A. Microglial nodule

   B. Abscess

   C. Secondary structure of Sherer

   D. Granuloma

   E. Vascular proliferation

93. (See Figure 92) The lesion in this case is associated with what tumor?

   A. Lymphoma

   B. Germinoma

   C. Meningioma

   D. Metastatic carcinoma

   E. Embryonal carcinoma

94. (See Figure 92) This tumor is most likely to arise in a(n)

   A. 59-yr-old male, frontal lobe

   B. 60-yr-old female, temporal lobe

   C. 14-yr-old male, pineal gland

   D. 15-yr-old female, pineal gland

   E. 82-yr-old male, pituitary gland

95. The lesion seen here represents a(n)

   A. Arteriovenous malformation

   B. Cavernous angioma

   C. Venous angioma

   D. Varix

   E. Capillary telangiectasia

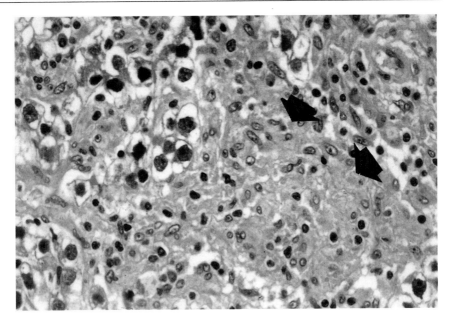

Questions 92, 93, and 94

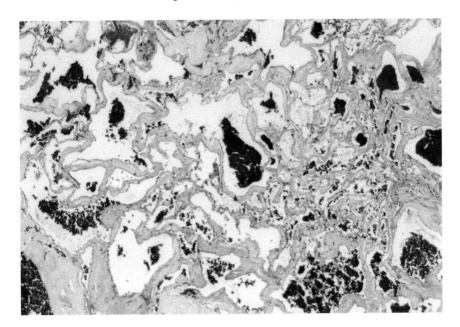

Question 95

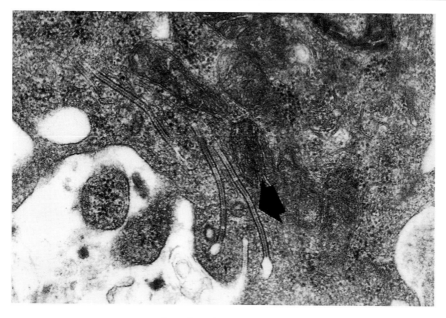

Questions 96, 97, and 98

96. The elongated structures (arrow) seen here represent

    A. Abnormal mitochondria

    B. Cilia

    C. Blepharoplasts

    D. Melanosomes

    E. Birbeck granules

97. (See Figure 96) The most likely diagnosis is

    A. Ependymoma

    B. Mitochondrial myopathy

    C. Melanoma

    D. Histiocytosis X

    E. Erdheim-Chester disease

98. (See Figure 96) The cells that contain these structures characteristically stain with antibody

    A. GFAP

    B. HMB-45

    C. CD3

    D. CD1a

    E. HAM 56

99. The organism seen here represents

    A. Amebiasis

    B. Cysticercosis

    C. Schistosomiasis

    D. Trypanosomiasis

    E. Toxoplasmosis

100. (See Figure 99) The organism causing this lesion is

    A. *Taenia solium*

    B. *Trypanosoma brucei*

    C. *Entamoeba histolytica*

    D. *Trichonella spiralis*

    E. *Iodamoeba buetschlii*

101. The pathology illustrated here represents

    A. Oligodendroglioma

    B. Astrocytoma

    C. Ependymoma

    D. Reactive astrocytosis

    E. Lymphoma

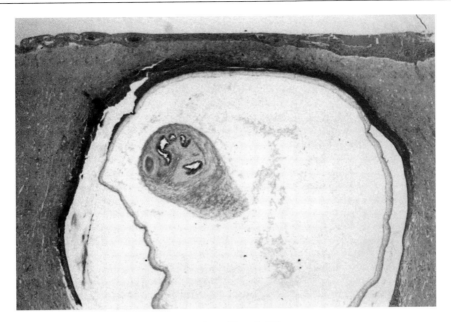

Questions 99 and 100

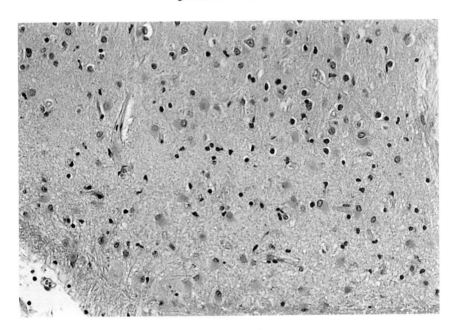

Question 101

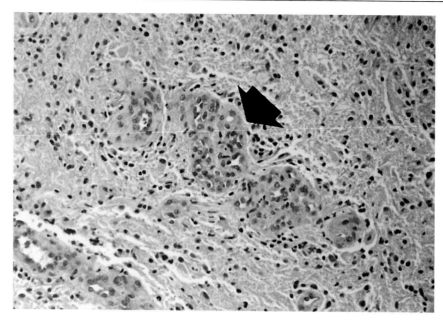

Questions 102 and 103

102. The structure denoted by the arrow represents

A. Secondary structure of Scherer

B. Vascular proliferation

C. Necrosis

D. Vascular invasion

E. None of the above

103. (See Figure 102) The lesion seen here in a 76-yr-old male represents a(n)

A. WHO grade I astrocytoma

B. WHO grade II astrocytoma

C. WHO grade III astrocytoma

D. WHO grade IV astrocytoma

E. Ependymoma

104. The photomicrograph here represents what normal structure?

A. Pineal gland

B. Leptomeninges

C. Pituitary adenohypophysis

D. Pituitary neurohypophysis

E. Pituitary pars intermedia

105. The area seen here is consistent with a(n)

A. Caudate nucleus

B. Hippocampus

C. Dentate nucleus

D. Olivary nucleus

E. None of the above

106. (See figure 105) The fascicles of myelinated fibers seen here (arrow) are referred to as

A. Lines of Baillarger

B. Stria of Gennari

C. Bundles of Wilson

D. Polymorphous bundles

E. None of the above

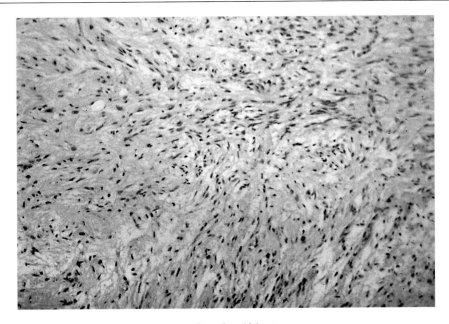

Question 104

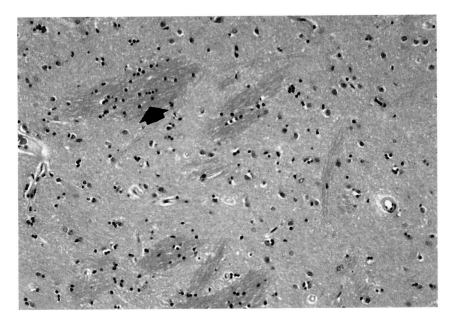

Questions 105 and 106

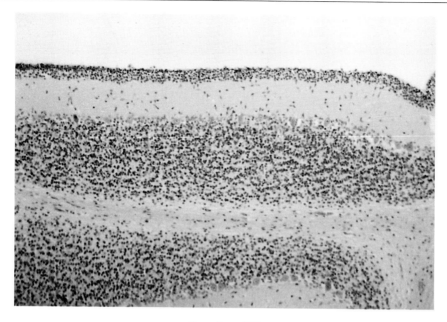

Questions 107

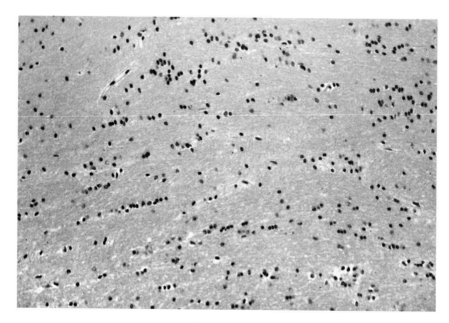

Question 108

107. The age of the patient here most likely is

A. 3 mo

B. 3 yr

C. 13 yr

D. 30 yr

E. 60 yr

108. The photomicrograph here was most likely taken from which location?

A. Frontal lobe cortex

B. Frontal lobe white matter

C. Caudate

D. Hippocampus

E. Pineal gland

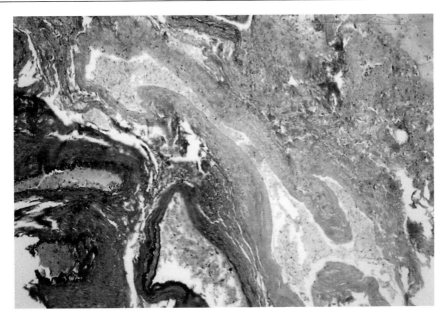

Question 109

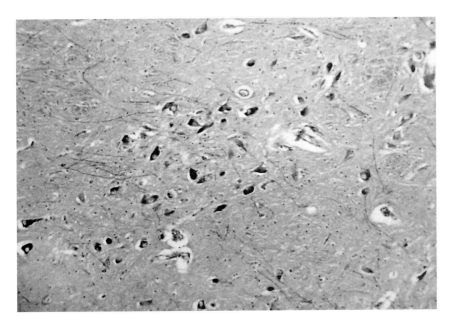

Question 110

109. The elastic stained section here represents a(n)

A. Arteriovenous malformation

B. Cavernous angioma

C. Venous angioma

D. Hemangioblastoma

E. Capillary telangiectasia

110. The melanin pigmented neurons seen here belong to which neuronal group?

A. Dentate nucleus

B. Substantia nigra

C. Hypoglossal nucleus

D. Red nucleus

E. Olivary nucleus

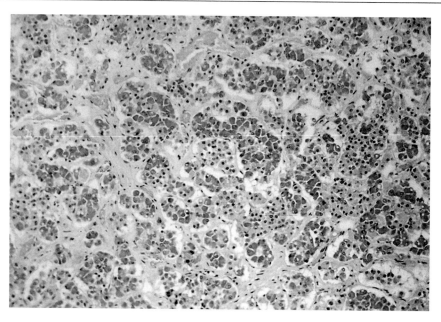

Question 111

111. What normal structure is represented here?

  A. Pineal gland

  B. Arachnoidal cap cells

  C. Choroid plexus

  D. Skeletal muscle

  E. None of the above

112. The mass seen here represents a(n)

  A. Astrocytoma

  B. Infarct

  C. Abscess

  D. Granuloma

  E. Demyelinating plaque

113. This 38-yr-old male has

  A. Non-Hodgkin's lymphoma

  B. Malaria

  C. Medulloblastoma

  D. Amebiasis

  E. Toxoplasmosis

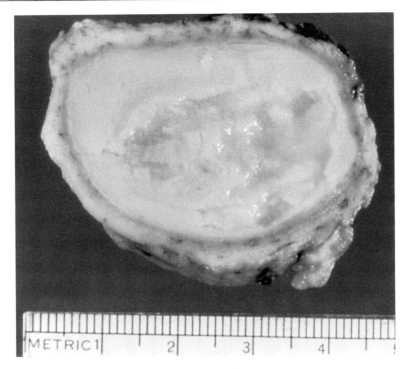

Question 112

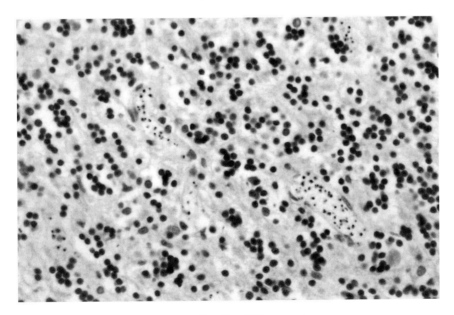

Question 113

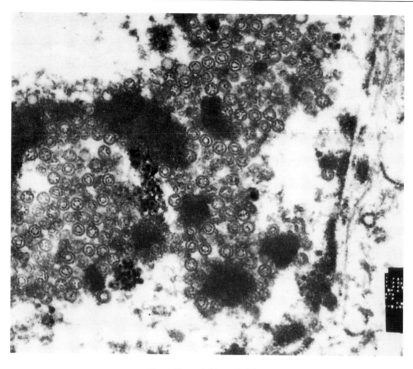

Questions 114 and 115

114. The organism seen here by electron microscopy represents

    A. Cytomegalovirus

    B. Toxoplasmosis

    C. Cryptococcus

    D. Progressive multifocal leukoencephalopathy

    E. *E. coli*

115. (See Figure 114) In an immunocompromised adult, the most common histologic manifestation of an infection by this organism is

    A. Granuloma

    B. Leptomeningitis

    C. Abscess

    D. Demyelination

    E. Microglial nodule

116. This luxol-fast blue stained section of periventricular tissue shows areas of decreased white matter staining in a 28-yr-old female. Cells that may be seen in these regions include all of the following except

    A. Reactive astrocytes

    B. Macrophages

    C. Neutrophils

    D. Lymphocytes

    E. Microglial cells

117. The findings in this lesion represent a(n)

    A. Contusion

    B. Acute infarct

    C. Subacute infarct

    D. Remote infarct

    E. Tumor

118. (See Figure 117) The most likely age of this lesion is

    A. 24 hr

    B. 48 hr

    C. 72 hr

    D. 5–7 d

    E. 3 mo

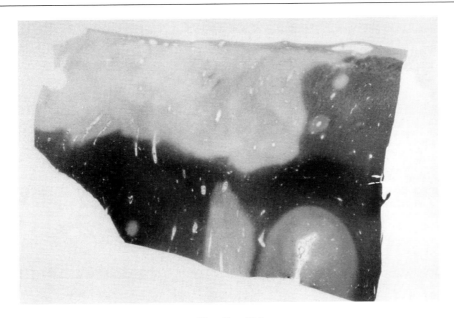

Question 116

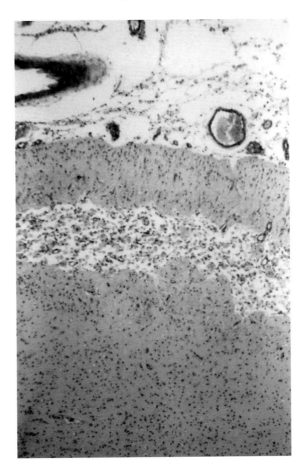

Questions 117 and 118

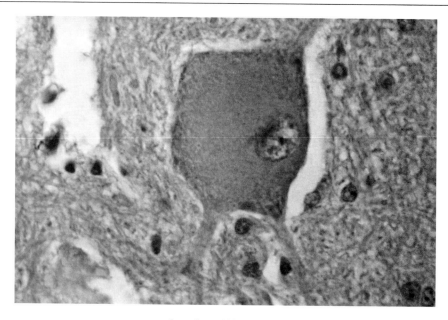

Questions 119 and 120

119. The cell shown here represents a(n)

A. Neuron

B. Astrocyte

C. Microglial cell

D. Oligodendroglial cell

E. Endothelial cell

120. (See Figure 119) The process shown in this cell represents

A. Ischemic changes

B. Central chromatolysis

C. Ferruginization

D. Neuronophagia

E. Creutzfeldt astrocyte

121. The section seen here is located where?

A. Frontal lobe cortex

B. Thalamus

C. Pons

D. Midbrain

E. Cerebellum

122. (See Figure 121) The changes seen in the large neurons is the result of

A. Ischemia

B. Central chromatolysis

C. Lipofuscin

D. Neuronophagia

E. Ferruginization

123. The accumulation of GM2 ganglioside material in these cells is characteristic of

A. Gaucher's disease

B. Tay-Sachs disease

C. Ceroid-lipofuscinosis

D. Hunter's disease

E. Leigh's disease

124. (See Figure 123) The cells in which the material has accumulated are

A. Astrocytes

B. Ependymal cells

C. Microglial cells

D. Neurons

E. Oligodendrocytes

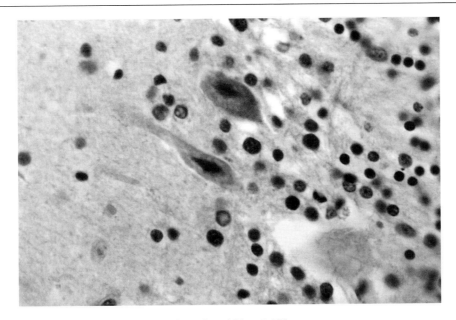

Questions 121 and 122

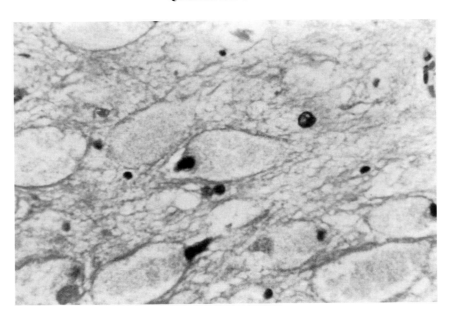

Questions 123 and 124

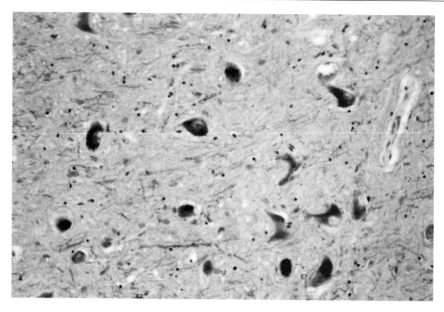

Question 125

125. The structure most likely to be encountered in these neurons in a patient with Parkinson's disease is

   A. Neuritic plaque

   B. Hirano body

   C. Lewy body

   D. Neurofibrillary tangle

   E. Granulovacuolar degeneration

126. The paler staining cells denoted by the arrow represent

   A. Purkinje cells

   B. Granular cells

   C. Lymphocytes

   D. Bergmann astrocytes

   E. Corpora amylacea

127. (See figure 126) All of the following conditions are likely to result in the pathology seen here except

   A. Chronic ischemic change

   B. Chronic epilepsy

   C. Alcoholism

   D. Infiltrating astrocytoma

   E. Dilantin toxicity

128. The patient is a 12-yr-old female with a recent measles infection. She now presents with seizures and dystonia. The diagnosis on biopsy is

   A. Oligodendroglioma

   B. Progressive multifocal leukoencephalopathy

   C. Subacute sclerosing panencephalitis

   D. Lymphoma

   E. None of the above

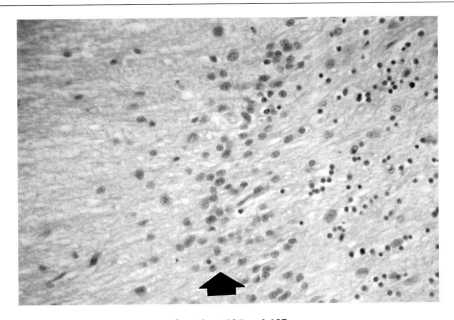

Questions 126 and 127

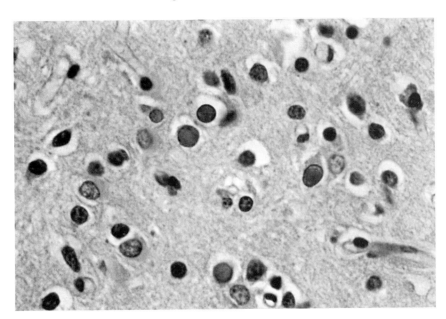

Question 128

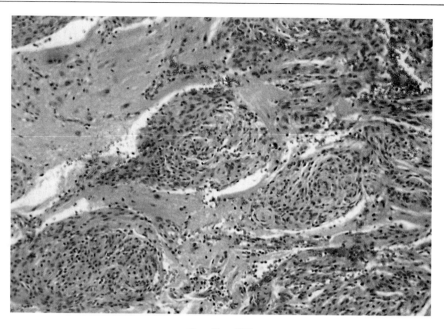

Question 129

129. The meningioma seen here is best classified as
    A. Syncytial
    B. Fibrous
    C. Invasive
    D. Metaplastic
    E. Rhabdoid

130. This infant has diffuse white matter abnormalities on imaging studies. The diagnosis is
    A. Alexander's disease
    B. Metachromatic leukodystrophy
    C. Globoid cell leukodystrophy
    D. Adrenoleukodystrophy
    E. Canavan's disease

131. (See Figure 130) The lesion seen is associated with a deficiency of
    A. Arylsulfatase A
    B. Galactocerebroside-B galactosidase
    C. Aspartoacylase
    D. Phospholipase
    E. None of the above

132. (See Figure 130) The pattern of inheritance associated with this condition is
    A. X-linked recessive
    B. Autosomal dominant
    C. Autosomal recessive
    D. Sporadic
    E. X-linked dominant

133. The changes seen here are most likely related to
    A. Fat emboli
    B. Methanol ingestion
    C. Kernicterus
    D. Ethanol toxicity
    E. Arsenic toxicity

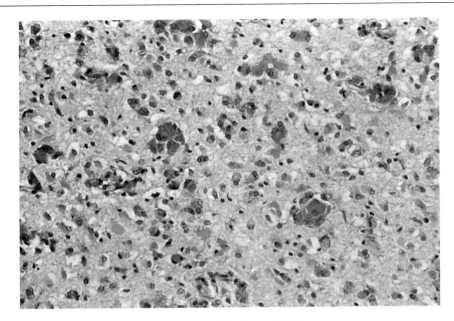

Questions 130, 131, and 132

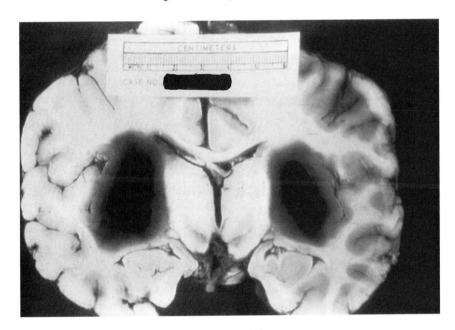

Question 133

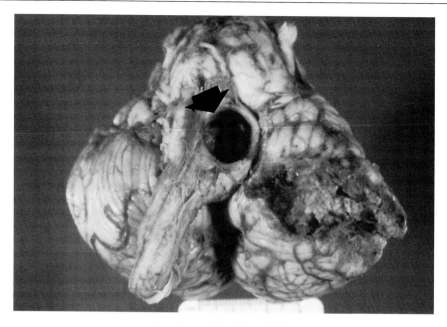

Questions 134, 135, and 136

134. The lesion denoted by the arrow is a(n)

    A. Arteriovenous malformation

    B. Air embolism

    C. Aneurysm

    D. Venous angioma

    E. Moyamoya disease

135. (See Figure 134) Microscopically, the defect that defines this lesion is

    A. A mixture of arterial and venous vessels

    B. Intimal fibroplasia

    C. Atherosclerosis

    D. Loss of arterial media

    E. Fragmented elastic lamina of the vessel wall

136. (See Figure 134) The other gross pathologic abnormality evident in this picture is

    A. Infarct

    B. Ganglioglioma

    C. Dandy-Walker syndrome

    D. Subdural hematoma

    E. Fat emboli

137. The lesion seen here most likely represents a(n)

    A. Vascular malformation

    B. Contusion

    C. Infarct

    D. Air embolism

    E. Aneurysm

138. The cell denoted by the arrow represents a(n)

    A. Reactive astrocyte

    B. Gemistocyte

    C. Creutzfeldt astrocyte

    D. Alzheimer type I astrocyte

    E. Alzheimer type II astrocyte

139. (See Figure 138) This cell is most likely to be encountered in the setting of

    A. Tumor

    B. Demylinating disease

    C. Diabetic encephalopathy

    D. Hepatic encephalopathy

    E. Progressive multifocal leukoencephalopathy

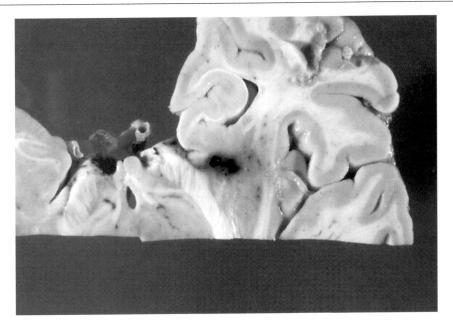

Question 137

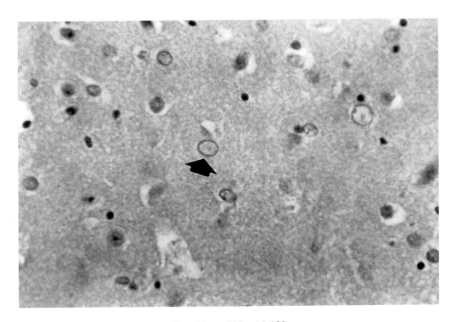

Questions 138 and 139

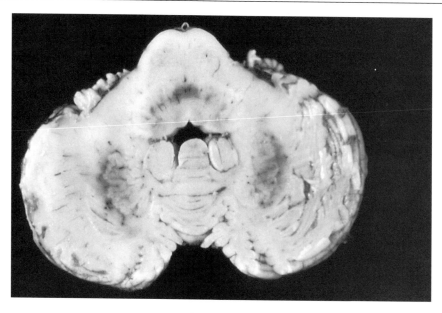

Question 140

140. The darker areas have a yellow coloration in this autopsy specimen from a 2-wk-old baby with a history of hemolytic anemia. The lesions seen represent
    A. Multifocal infarcts
    B. Hemorrhage
    C. Bilirubin encephalopathy
    D. Fetal alcoholism syndrome
    E. Ponto-subicular necrosis

141. The changes seen here are the result of
    A. Atrophy
    B. Edema
    C. Polymicrogyria
    D. Subarachnoid hemorrhage
    E. Lissencephaly

142. The lesion seen here represents a(n)
    A. Vascular malformation
    B. Acute infarct
    C. Remote infarct
    D. Multiple sclerosis plaque
    E. Lacunar infarct

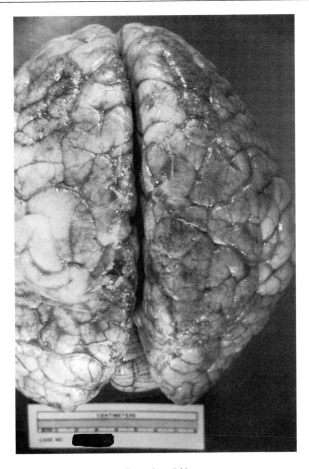

Question 141

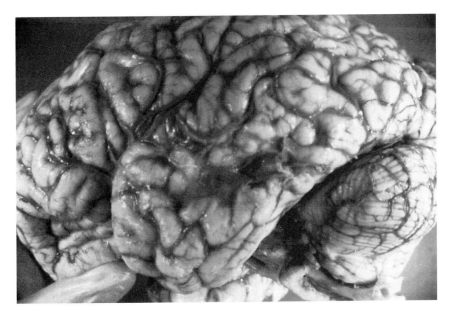

Question 142

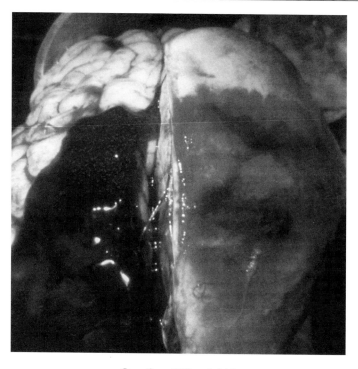

Questions 143 and 144

143. The most accurate diagnosis here is

    A. Contusion

    B. Epidural hematoma

    C. Subdural hematoma

    D. Arteriovenous malformation

    E. Meningitis

144. (See Figure 143) The lesion seen here is gener-
    ally associated with the rupture of which vessel?

    A. Middle meningeal artery

    B. Bridging veins

    C. Vertebral artery

    D. Sagittal sinus

    E. Middle cerebral artery

145. The changes seen here are most consistent with

    A. Atherosclerotic vasculopathy

    B. Moyamoya syndrome

    C. Binswanger's disease

    D. CADASIL

    E. Amyloid angiopathy

146. (See Figure 145) The gene defect associated with
    this lesion is located at chromosome

    A. It is not associated with a gene defect

    B. 22

    C. 19

    D. 14

    E. 3

147. The lesion shown here in this 62-yr-old female
    represents a(n)

    A. Demyelinative plaque

    B. Laminar infarct

    C. Pseudolaminar infarct

    D. Abscess

    E. Creutzfeldt-Jakob disease

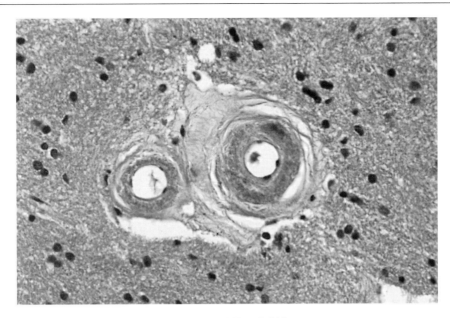

Questions 145 and 146

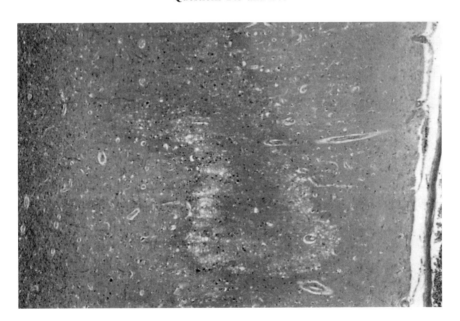

Question 147

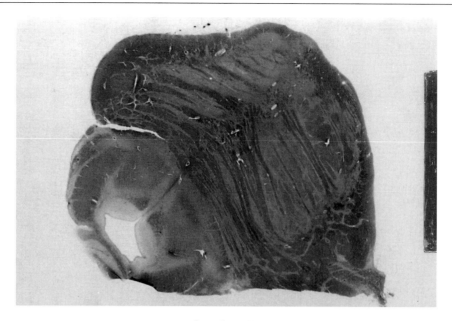

Question 148

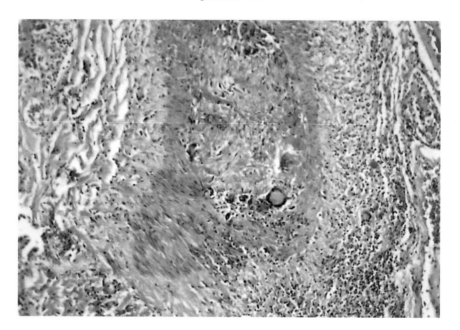

Question 149

148. The changes seen here are most likely related to
    A. Brain stem glioma
    B. Syringobulbia
    C. Degeneration of corticospinal tracts
    D. Chiari malformation
    E. Olivopontocerebellar atrophy

149. The changes seen in this vessel are most likely the result of
    A. Lymphoma
    B. Polyarteritis nodosa
    C. Granulomatous angiitis
    D. Hypersensitivity angiitis
    E. Amyloid angiopathy

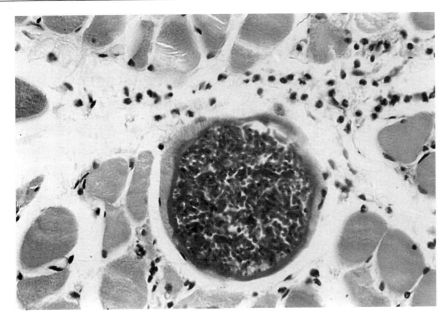

Question 150

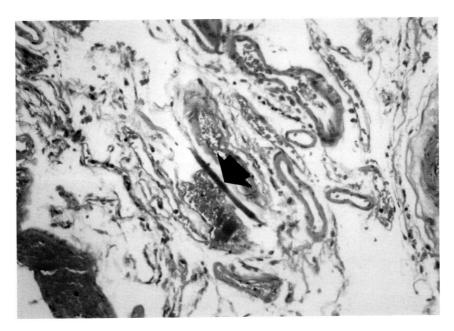

Question 151

150. The organisms seen here represent
    A. Trichinosis
    B. Cysticercosis
    C. Trypanosomiasis
    D. Sarcocystis
    E. Toxoplasmosis

151. The leptomeningeal organism denoted by the arrow represents
    A. Schistosomiasis
    B. Malaria
    C. Cysticercosis
    D. Echinococcus
    E. Strongyloides

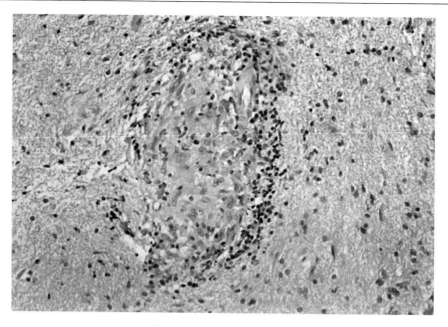

Questions 152, 153, and 154

152. The lesion seen here represents a(n)

   A. Granuloma

   B. Microglial nodule

   C. Hamartoma

   D. Thrombus

   E. Vascular proliferation

153. (See Figure 152) Stains that may be useful in further delineating the etiology of this lesion would include

   A. GMS and PAS

   B. GMS and fite

   C. GFAP and GMS

   D. GFAP and fite

   E. GFAP and Ziehl-Neelson

154. (See Figure 152) The lesion seen here may be encountered in all of the following conditions except

   A. Listeriosis

   B. Sarcoidosis

   C. Tuberculosis

   D. Wegener's vasculitis

   E. Germinoma

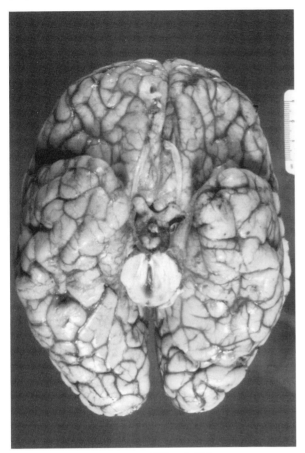

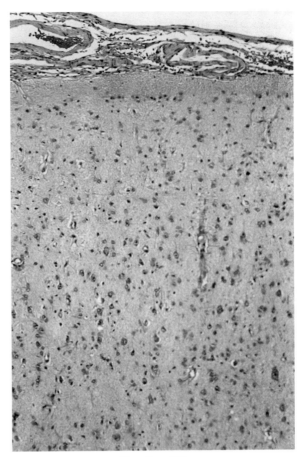

Questions 155 and 156   **Question 157**

155. The midbrain lesion seen here represents

   A. Vascular malformation

   B. Duret hemorrhage

   C. Diffuse axonal injury

   D. Fat emboli

   E. Lacunar infarct

156. (See Figure 155) The midbrain lesion is often seen associated with what other condition?

   A. Uncal herniation

   B. Central herniation

   C. Subfalcial herniation

   D. Tonsillar herniation

   E. Upward herniation

157. The abnormality shown in this cortical section from a 14-yr-old with chronic epilepsy represents

   A. No abnormality

   B. Cortical dysplasia

   C. Ganglioglioma

   D. Dysembryoplastic neuroepithelial tumor

   E. Pleomorphic xanthoastrocytoma

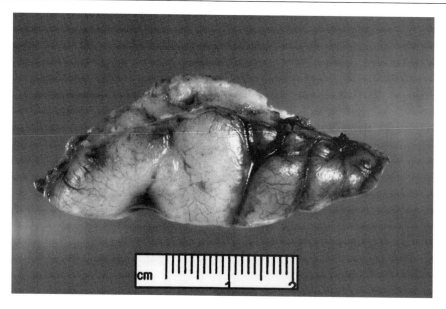

Question 158

158. This partial lobectomy specimen is from a 12-yr-old with tuberous sclerosis. The diagnosis is

   A. Subependymal giant-cell astrocytoma

   B. Cortical tuber

   C. Metastatic rhabdomyoma

   D. Lymphoma

   E. Hemangioblastoma

159. The findings in this myelin-stained section of spinal cord are most consistent with

   A. Thiamine deficiency

   B. Wilson's disease

   C. Menke's disease

   D. Subacute combined degeneration

   E. Herpes myelitis

160. The findings seen here are consistent with

   A. Infarct

   B. Mesial temporal sclerosis

   C. Anaplastic astrocytoma

   D. Carbon monoxide toxicity

   E. Wernicke encephalopathy

161. (See Figure 160) The underlying cause of the pathology seen here is

   A. Poor cerebral perfusion

   B. Not known

   C. Vitamin deficiency

   D. Possibly suicide related

   E. A risk from prior radiation therapy

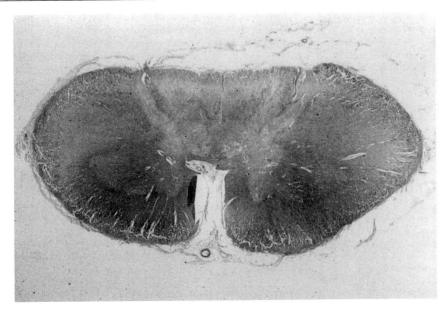

Question 159

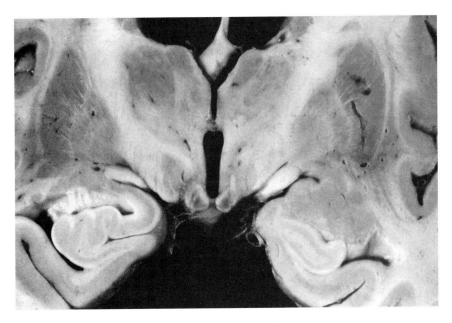

Questions 160 and 161

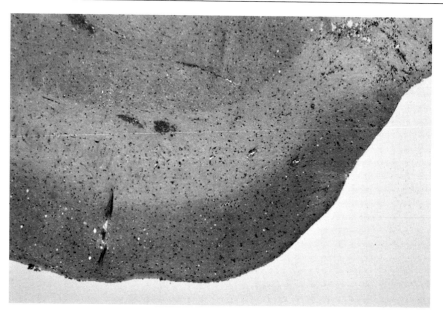

Question 162

162. The changes in the hippocampus of this 8-yr-old with intractable seizures is the result of

    A. Hippocampal sclerosis

    B. Cortical dysplasia

    C. Ganglioglioma

    D. Cortical tuber

    E. Neuronal heterotopia

163. The changes seen in the leptomeninges in this 68-yr-old male with bacterial meningitis represent

    A. Granuloma formation

    B. Abscess

    C. Vasculitis with thrombosis

    D. Infarct

    E. Hemorrhage

164. The GFAP immunostain seen here is highlighting what cells?

    A. Ependymal cells

    B. Astrocytes

    C. Microglial cells

    D. Oligodendroglial cells

    E. Neurons

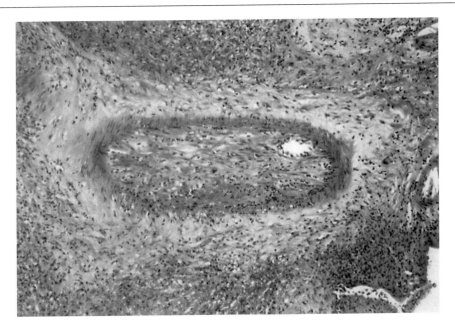

Question 163

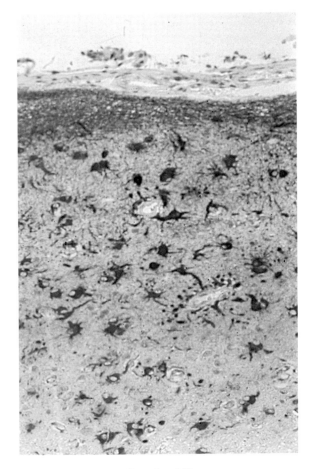

Question 164

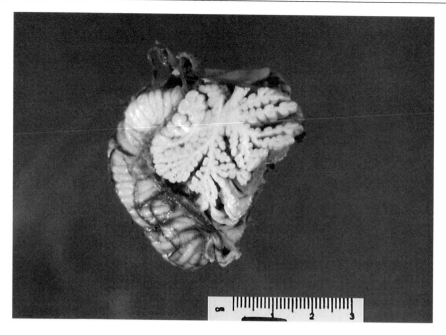

Question 165

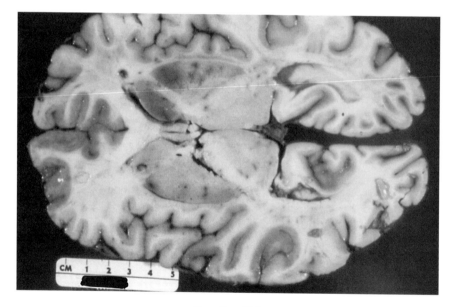

Question 166

165. The findings here are most likely related to
    A. Infarct
    B. Ethanol
    C. Carbon monoxide
    D. Aluminum toxicity
    E. Manganese toxicity

166. The pathology seen here in this 48-yr-old male with endocarditis and atrial fibrillation most likely represents
    A. Demyelinating disease
    B. Embolic acute infarcts
    C. Air embolism
    D. Multiple organizing abscesses
    E. Storage disease

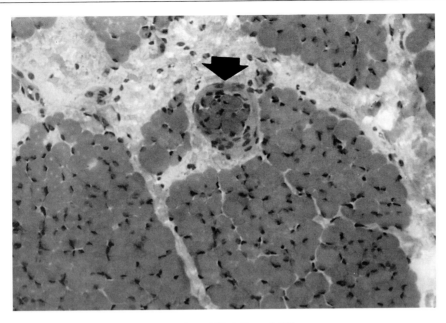

Questions 167, 168, and 169

167. The structure denoted by the arrow represents a
    A. Muscle fascicle
    B. Neuromuscular junction
    C. Muscle spindle
    D. Blood vessel
    E. Sarcomeric unit

168. (See Figure 167) This biopsy is from a 3-mo-old with hypotonia and tongue fasciculations. The diagnosis is
    A. Werdnig-Hoffmann disease
    B. Central core disease
    C. Duchenne dystrophy
    D. Centronuclear myopathy
    E. Pompe's diease

169. (See Figure 167) All of the following are likely pathologic findings in this patient except
    A. Scattered type I hypertrophy
    B. Loss of neurons in Onuf's nucleus
    C. Increased muscle spindles
    D. Atrophy of anterior spinal roots
    E. Fascicular atrophy of the muscle

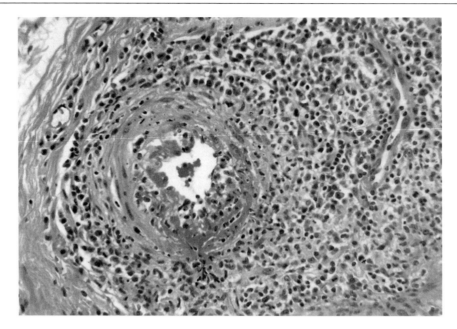

Question 170

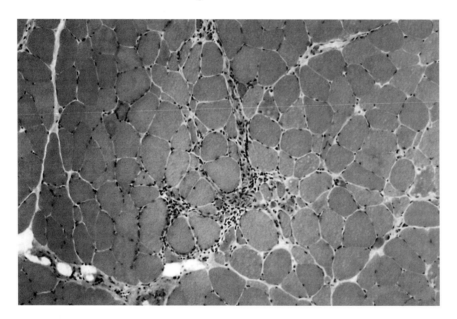

Question 171

170. The vessel seen here from a vastus lateralis muscle biopsy shows changes diagnostic of

   A. Necrotizing vasculitis

   B. Inclusion body myositis

   C. Trichinosis

   D. Dermatomyositis

   E. Polymyositis

171. The changes in the biopsy are most consistent
with a diagnosis of

   A. Polymyositis

   B. Dermatomyositis

   C. Neurogenic atrophy

   D. Vasculitis

   E. Acid maltase deficiency

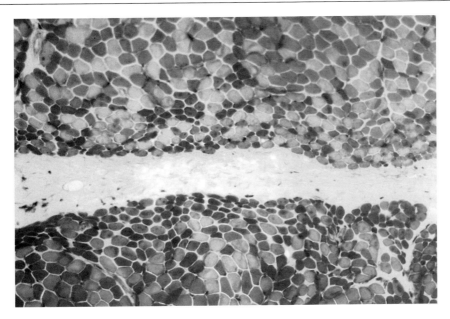

Questions 172 and 173

172. The pathologic findings on the ATPase pH 4.6 stain are suggestive of

    A. Dermatomyositis

    B. Neurogenic atrophy

    C. Muscular dystrophy

    D. Inclusion body myositis

    E. Spinal muscular atrophy

173. (See Figure 172) All of the following are associated with this disease process except

    A. Arthralgia

    B. Calcinosis

    C. Steroid resistance

    D. Malignancy

    E. Non-necrotizing vasculitis

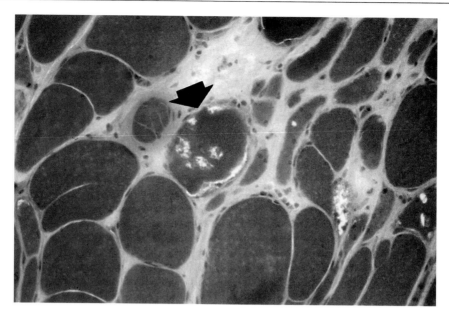

Questions 174 and 175

174. The structures observed in the myofiber denoted
    by the arrow on this Gomori trichrome stain
    represent

    A. A freeze artifact

    B. Glycogen storage material

    C. Rimmed vacuoles

    D. Nemaline rods

    E. Viral inclusions

175. (See Figure 174) The presence of this finding in
    the setting of an inflammatory myopathic biopsy
    is highly suggestive of

    A. Angiopathic polymyositis

    B. Viral myositis

    C. Fungal myositis

    D. Inclusion body myositis

    E. Myasthenia gravis

176. The NADH-stained section shown reveals

    A. Ring fibers

    B. Moth-eaten fibers

    C. Target fibers

    D. Targetoid fibers

    E. Core fibers

177. (See Figure 176) This change is a common fea-
    ture observed in

    A. Polymyositis

    B. Neurogenic atrophy

    C. Myotonic dystrophy

    D. Mitochondrial myopathy

    E. Chloroquine myopathy

178. On this ATPase-stained section, the dark staining
    fibers are

    A. Type I

    B. Type IIA

    C. Type IIB

    D. Type IIC

    E. Type III

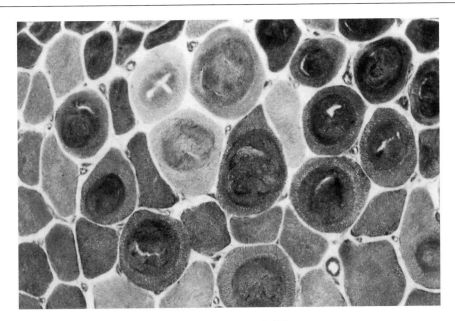

Questions 176 and 177

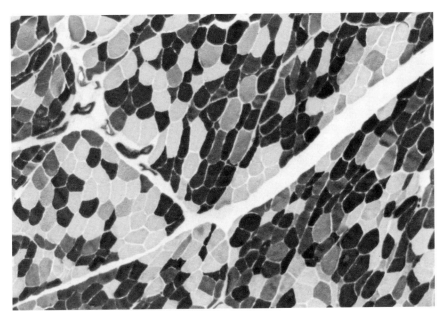

Question 178

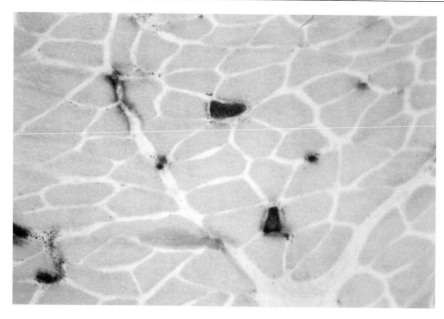

Question 179

179. The positive staining on this alkaline phosphatase stain represents

    A. Degenerating fibers

    B. Regenerating fibers

    C. Acutely denervated fibers

    D. Ragged red fibers

    E. A mitochondrial defect

180. The fibrillary structures observed within the nucleus of this myocyte are characteristic of what entity?

    A. Mitochondrial myopathy

    B. Inclusion body myositis

    C. Glycogen storage disease

    D. Amyloid

    E. A parasite

181. (See Figure 180) The structure denoted by the arrow represents a(n)

    A. I band

    B. A band

    C. H band

    D. M band

    E. Z band

182. The vacuolar structures seen here likely represent

    A. Glycogen storage disease

    B. Lipid storage disease

    C. Mitochondrial degeneration

    D. Core formations

    E. A freeze artifact

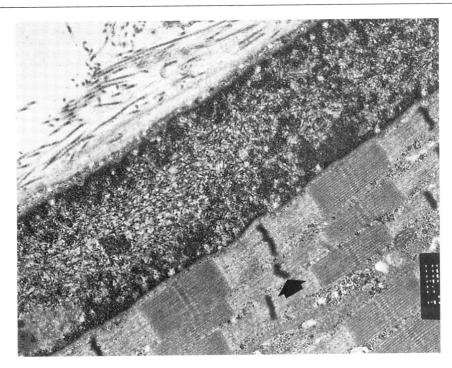

Questions 180 and 181

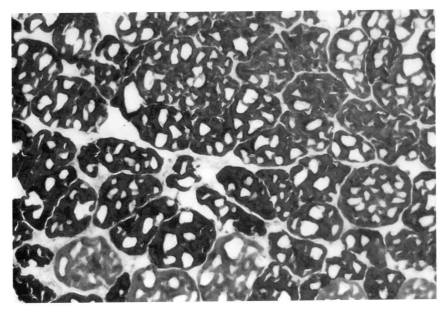

Question 182

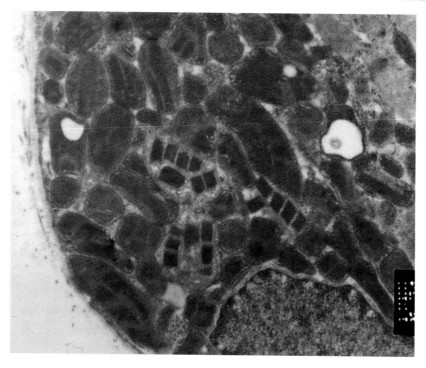

Questions 183 and 184

183. The abnormality seen ultrastructurally represents an abnormality of

    A. T system

    B. Mitochondria

    C. Sarcoplasmic reticulum

    D. Ribosomes

    E. Golgi

184. (See Figure 183) The abnormality seen here is most commonly associated with

    A. Amyloid deposition

    B. Ragged red fibers

    C. Autophagic vacuoles

    D. Core fibers

    E. Nemaline rods

185. The absence of staining on this cytochrome oxidase stain is indicative of a possible

    A. Glycogen storage disease

    B. Lipid storage disease

    C. Viral infection

    D. Mitochondrial myopathy

    E. None of the above

186. The curvilinear bodies seen here ultrastructurally are most commonly associated with

    A. Mitochondrial encephalomyopathy

    B. Ceroid lipofuscinosis

    C. Lafora body disease

    D. Globoid cell leukodystrophy

    E. Metachromatic leukodystrophy

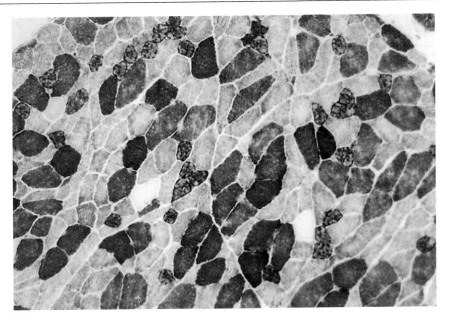

Question 185

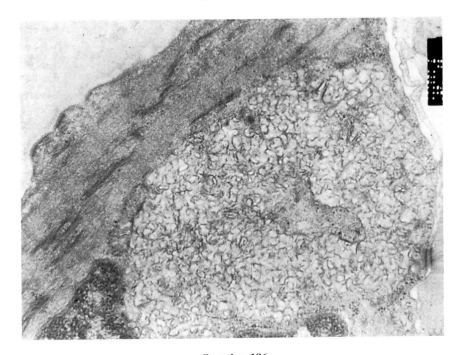

Question 186

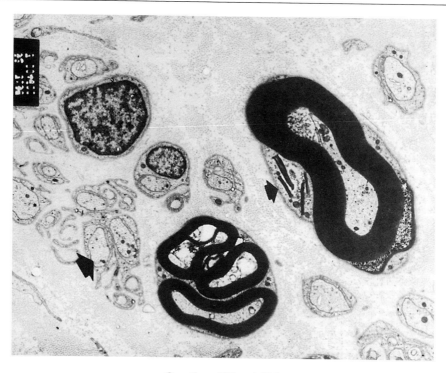

Questions 187 and 188

187. The cystalloid structures denoted by the small
arrow represent

 A. Renaut bodies

 B. Myelin

 C. Schmidt-Lanterman clefts

 D. Pi granules of Reich

 E. Corpuscles of Erzholz

188. (See Figure 187) The structure denoted on the
left by the larger arrow is a(n)

 A. Schwann cell

 B. Collagen

 C. Unmyelinated axon

 D. Myelinated axon

 E. Renaut body

189. The finely fibrillar material (arrow) in the wall of
this epineurial vessel stains positively with Congo
red. The best diagnosis is

 A. Vasculitic neuropathy

 B. CADASIL

 C. Amyloid neuropathy

 D. Adrenoleukodystrophy

 E. Porphyria

190. (See Figure 189) The most common mutation
associated with the hereditary form of this condition involves what gene?

 A. Thyroglobulin

 B. Notch 3

 C. Transthyretin

 D. Notch 5

 E. None of the above

191. The arrow corresponds to a(n)

 A. Schwann cell nucleus

 B. Endothelial cell

 C. Fibroblast

 D. Mast cell

 E. Renaut body

192. (See Figure 191) The pathology seen here is most
likely to be encountered in the setting of

 A. Traumatic neuroma

 B. Amyloid neuropathy

 C. Vasculitic neuropathy

 D. Charcot-Marie-Tooth disease

 E. Thiamine deficiency neuropathy

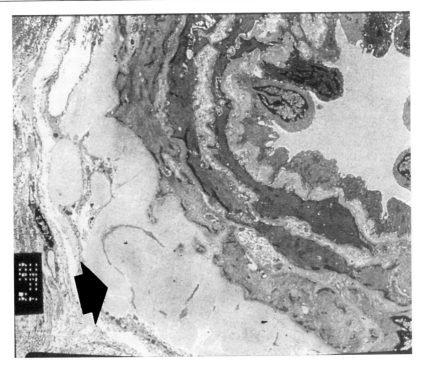

Questions 189 and 190

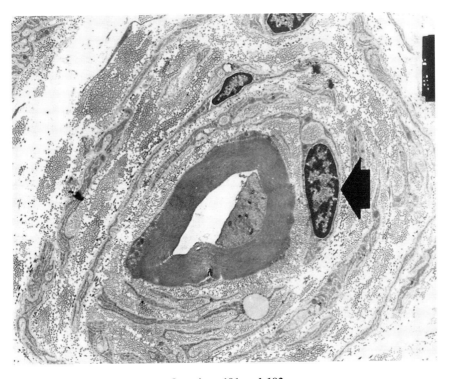

Questions 191 and 192

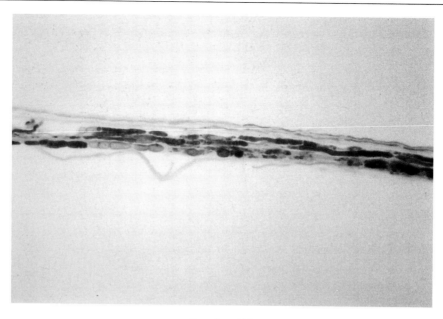

Question 193

193. The changes seen in this teased nerve preparation most likely would be seen in

   A. Vasculitic neuropathy

   B. Charcot-Marie-Tooth disease

   C. Guillain-Barre syndrome

   D. CIDP

   E. Diphtheritic neuropathy

194. The change seen here represents

   A. Axonal sprouting

   B. Demyelination

   C. Remyelination

   D. Onion bulb formation

   E. Renaut body

195. This muscle is from an 8-yr-old male who is wheelchair bound. The most likely diagnosis is

   A. Polymyositis

   B. Dermatomyostitis

   C. Duchenne muscular dystrophy

   D. Myotonic muscular dystrophy

   E. Becker muscular dystrophy

196. (See Figure 195) Confirmation of the diagnosis in this case would involve

   A. T-cell subset analysis

   B. Serology testing for ANA

   C. Sedimentation rate

   D. Dystrophin analysis

   E. Emerin analysis

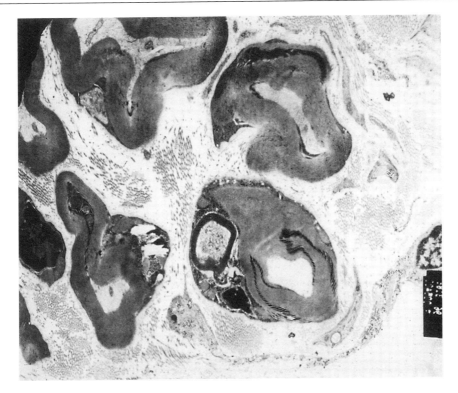

Question 194

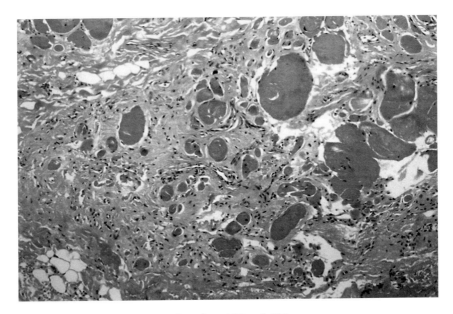

Questions 195 and 196

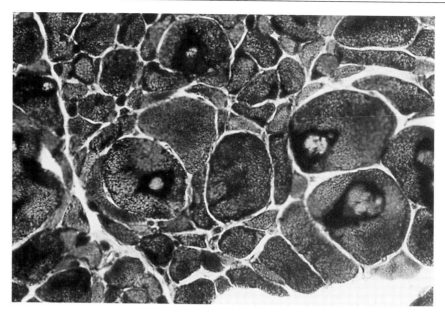

Questions 197 and 198

197. The lesions seen on this NADH stain represent
     A. Moth-eaten fibers
     B. Rimmed vacuoles
     C. Nemaline rods
     D. Target fibers
     E. Targetoid fibers

198. (See Figure 197) This biopsy is most likely to be seen in the setting of
     A. Myasthenia gravis
     B. Lambert-Eaton syndrome
     C. Werdnig-Hoffman disease
     D. Neurogenic atrophy
     E. Polymyositis

199. The pattern of atrophy observed here is suggestive of
     A. Dermatomyositis
     B. Spinal muscular atrophy
     C. Inclusion body myositis
     D. Steroid myopathy
     E. Diabetic neuropathy-associated neurogenic atrophy

200. The vacuoles seen here stain with acid phosphatase and are filled with PAS-positive material. The diagnosis is
     A. Carnitine deficiency
     B. Myophosphorylase deficiency
     C. Acid maltase deficiency
     D. Succinate dehydrogenase deficiency
     E. Phosphofructokinase deficiency

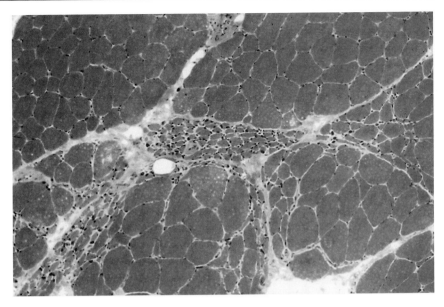

Question 199

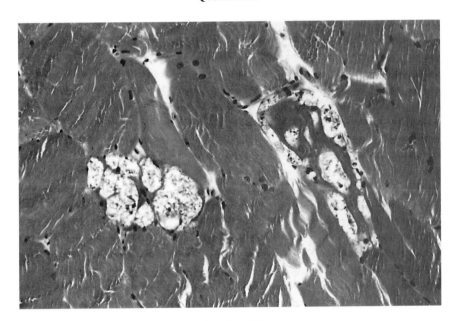

Question 200

13 Answers to Figures with Questions

1. A (Chapter 5.III.A)   The plexiform neurofibroma is almost exclusively seen in the setting of neurofibromatosis type I.

2. E (Chapter 3.IV.A)   Dural-based meningioma, the most commonly encountered cytogenetic abnormality is a deletion associated with chromosome 22.

3. C (Chapter 3.I.F)   Perinecrotic pseudopalisading in a glioblastoma multiforme.

4. B(chapter 3 I L)   Subependymal giant-cell astrocytoma arising in the setting of tuberous sclerosis.

5. A (Chapter 1.I.B)   Rosenthal fibers in a pilocytic astrocytoma.

6. D (Chapter 3.VIII.A)   Angiotropic large cell lymphomas frequently are CD20 positive (B-cell immunophenotype) and are typically confined to vascular lumina.

7. C (Chapter 3.X.C)   The mixture of large "germ" cells and lymphocytes is characteristic of germinoma.

8. D (Chapter 3.VII.D)   The haphazard proliferation of peripheral neural tissue with collagen in the arm is best designated as traumatic neuroma.

9. A (Chapter 5.I.D)   The absence of convolution seen in this brain is characteristic of lissencephaly (agyria).

10. C (Chapter 3.IV.A)   The tumor shown is marked by cells arranged in a whorled configuration, characteristic of a syncytial or meningotheliomatous meningioma.

11. D (Chapter 1.I.G)   A meningioma with numerous laminated calcifications known as psammoma bodies.

12. A (Chapter 5.III.A)   Meningoangiomatosis is characterized by a perivascular proliferation of meningothelial cells and is associated with neurofibromatosis type I.

13. C (Chapter 3.X.G)   Squamous cell carcinoma with large keratinized epithelial-appearing cells infiltrating dura.

14. C (Chapter 3.II.E)   The location, appearance, and immunohistochemical profile are classic for central neurocytoma.

15. B (Chapter 3.VII.A)   The nuclear palisading (Verocay bodies) and mixed compact (Antoni A) and loose regions (Antoni B) are characteristic of a schwannoma.

16. A (Chapter 3.IV.B)   The presence of vacuolated epithelioid cells (physaliphorous) in a bone-based sacrococcygeal mass is suggestive of a chordoma.

17. B (Chapter 3.VI.C)   The structure denoted by the arrow is a Homer Wright pseudorosette in a medulloblastoma.

18. C (Chapter 3.VI.C)   The cells seen are from a medulloblastoma.

19. B (Chapter 4.II.H)   The lesion shown here (porencephaly) is usually the result of an ischemic/infarct event.

20. E (Chapter 7.I.B)   The zebra bodies seen by electron microscopy are a common findings in Tay-Sachs disease.

21. B (Chapter 5.I.F)   The lesion seen represents a partial agenesis of the corpus callosum.

22. D (Chapter 3.III.B)   The well-demarcated appearance of this intramedullary spinal cord mass is more commonly seen with ependymoma versus an astrocytoma.

23. C (Chapter 5.III.C)   The subependymal giant-cell astrocytoma seen here is associated with tuberous sclerosis.

24. A (Chapter 3.X.A)   The nested architectural pattern (zellballen), chromogranin positivity, and location are classic for paraganglioma.

25. A (Chapter 3.II.A)   The most common site of origin for oligodendroglioma is frontal lobe (it has the most white matter).

26. D (Chapter 3.I.N)   The lesion depicted here (asymmetrial enlargement of the brain stem) is most consistent with a brain stem glioma.

27. B (Chapter 3.X.D)   Adamantinomatous pattern of a craniopharyngioma.

28. A (Chapter 3.IX.A)   The location and appearance of the mass is most consistent with a colloid cyst of the third ventricle.

29. D (Chapter 3.V.A)   The lateral ventricle is the most likely location of choroid plexus papillomas arising in childhood.

30. C (Chapter 3.X.G)   The sharp interface between tumor and brain parenchyma and immunohistochemical profile is most consistent with melanoma (most glioblastoma multiforme show cross-immunoreactivity with cytokeratin AE1/3).

31. E (Chapter 5.III.B)   Bilateral acoustic schwannomas are diagnostic of neurofibromatosis type II, which is related to a chromosome 22 abnormality.

32. A (Chapter 3.X.E)   The most common secreting pituitary adenoma is a prolactinoma.

33. B (Chapter 5.I.D)   Polymicrogyria, seen in the figure, is associated with Zellweger's syndrome, a peroxisome abnormality.

34. A (Chapter 5.II.I)   The germinal matrix hemorrhage is most likely to occur in the premature infant.

35. E (Chapter 5.I.F)   The defect seen represents cavum septi pellucidi.

36. B (Chapter 3.III.B)   The cilia and ciliary body attachments are characteristic ultrastructural features of ependymoma.

37. A (Chapter 3.I.M)   The histologic appearance (pleomorphic astrocytic cells), clinical presentation, and low rate of cell proliferation are most consistent with a pleomorphic xanthoastrocytoma.

38. C (Chapter 3.I.H)   The gliosarcoma consists of reticulin-rich sarcomatous areas and GFAP-positive glioblastomatous areas.

39. B (Chapter 5.I.B)   The changes seen are most characteristic of a Chiari malformation.

40. D (Chapter 5.I.A)   Congenital dilatation of the central canal is termed hydromyelia.

41. E (Chapter 5.III.A)   The axillary freckling and café-au-lait macule are features of neurofibromatosis type I. All the listed lesions may be seen in this setting except subependymal giant cell astrocytoma (a feature of tuberous sclerosis).

42. A (Chapter 3.I.B)   Obliteration of the gray–white junction is a gross feature of infiltrating gliomas (in this case astrocytoma).

43. B (Chapter 3.II.A)   About 2% of oligodendrogliomas present with evidence of hemorrhage.

44. C (Chapter 3.I.F)   The gross appearance is most consistent with a glioblastoma multiforme.

45. C (Chapter 3.III.E)   The lesion depicted represents a myxopapillary ependymoma.

46. B (Chapter 6.I.D)   Multiple white matter lesions marked by reactive astrocytes, macrophages, and perivascular lymphocytes are suggestive of multiple sclerosis.

47. A (Chapter 6.II.D)   Numerous Rosenthal fibers in the setting of diffuse demyelination and megalencephaly are suggestive of Alexander's disease.

48. D (Chapter 3.III.D)   Subependymomas are marked by loose clustering of cell nuclei arranged against a fibrillary background. Microcystic change is fairly common.

49. D (Chapter 6.I.D)   Periventricular white matter plaques are a characteristic feature of multiple sclerosis.

50. D (Chapter 1.I.H)   The Sommer sector (CA1) region is denoted by the arrow.

51. B (Chapter 8.III.C)   The changes seen are characteristic of atrophy—ventricular dilatation, narrowing of gyri, widening of sulci. This patient had Alzheimer's disease.

52. A (Chapter 2.II.C)   The partially cavitated lesion denoted by the small arrow represents a remote infarct.

53. D (Chapter 1.I.H)   The large arrow is pointing at a normal appearing pineal gland.

54. E (Chapter 1.I.E)   The cell characterized by an elongated nucleus and scant cytoplasm represents a microglial cell.

55. C (Chapter 9.V.A)   The smaller arrow is pointing at a Toxoplasma gondii cyst.

56. C (Chapter 9.V.A) Rarely, microglial nodules, as seen here, are associated with Toxoplasmosis infection.

57. B (Chapter 9.IV.M) Multiple white matter lesions in an immunocompromised individual should raise the possibility of PML as a diagnosis.

58. D (Chapter 9.IV.L) The Cowdry A nuclear inclusions seen here are most characteristic of CMV infection.

59. B (Chapter 9.IV.L) The viral inclusions are associated with the ependymal lining present and ventricular space representing a ventriculitis.

60. D (Chapter 9.III.E) The broad-branching, nonseptate hyphae seen here are characteristic of Mucormycosis.

61. E (Chapter 9.III.E) Fusarium hyphae are morphologically similar to Aspergillus in tissue sections.

62. E (Chapter 9.VI.B) The clinical history and pathology (cortical spongiform degeneration with neuronal loss) are characteristic of Creutzfeldt-Jakob disease.

63. C (Chapter 9.VI.B) The star-burst-like structure represents a kuru plaque.

64. D (Chapter 1.I.B) The structure represents corpora amylacea, a laminated basophilic polyglucosan body associated with astrocytic foot processes.

65. B (Chapter 8.III.G) The granules with a clear halo represent granulovacuolar degeneration.

66. A (Chapter 8.III.G) Granulovacuolar degeneration is most likely to be seen in the setting of Alzheimer's disease.

67. A (Chapter 6.I.D) The periventricular areas of demyelination (plaques) is characteristic of multiple sclerosis.

68. B (Chapter 9.III.D) Dichotomously branching septate hyphae is characteristic of Aspergillus.

69. B (Chapter 3.III.B) The presence of true ependymal rosettes and perivascular pseudorosettes in this tumor is characteristic of an ependymoma.

70. C (Chapter 8.III.F) The structures seen here represent neuritic plaques.

71. A (Chapter 8.III.F) A Bodian stain will highlight the neuritic component of the plaque and a Congo red will stain the amyloid core.

72. B (Chapter 9.III.B) The thick mucopolysaccharide wall of Cryptococcus stains with mucicarmine.

73. A (Chapter 9.V.B) The organism seen represents Amebiasis in a background of necrosis.

74. A (Chapter 9.II.C) The cocci seen here most likely represent Meningococcus.

75. B (Chapter 9.IV.A) The large intranuclear viral inclusions seen here represent Cowdry type A inclusions.

76. B (Chapter 9.IV.M) Alzheimer type I astrocytes are a common finding in progressive multifocal leukoencephaly (result of JC virus infection)

77. B (Chapter 1.I.A) The intracytoplasmic material in many of the neurons here represents lipofuscin or aging pigment.

78. E (Chapter 9 IV I) The intraneuronal cytoplasmic Negri body is characteristic of rabies.

79. C (Chapter 8.III.E) The neuronal cytoplasmic silver positive structure represents a neurofibrillary tangle.

80. D (Chapter 8.III.E) Neurofibrillary tangles are not found in Herpes encephalitis.

81. B (Chapter 9.II.C) Herniation is not evident in this case. The brain is edematous and demonstrates vascular congestion and meningeal cloudiness consistent with a purulent meningitis.

82. D (Chapter 9.II.C) Secondary glioma development is not associated with purulent meningitis.

83. D (Chapter 9.II.C) *Streptococcus pneumoniae* is the most likely cause of community acquired bacterial meningitis in the elderly.

84. A (Chapter 1.I.F) The structure shown represents a normal choroid plexus, marked by fibrovascular cores lined by epithelioid cells.

85. C (Chapter 1.I.A) The cell shown represents a neuron.

86. B (Chapter 1.I.A) Neurons are most likely to stain with antibody to synaptophysin.

87. A (Chapter 2.V.A) Hypertension is the most common cause of nontraumatic intracerebral hemorrhage.

88. E (Chapter 5.III.D) Leptomeningeal venous angioma is a common finding in Sturge-Weber disease.

89. E (Chapter 5.III.D) There is no pattern of inheritance associated with Sturge-Weber disease.

90. B (Chapter 2.IV.B) The lesion illustrated represents an arteriovenous malformation that has been embolized.

91. C (Chapter 9.IV.M) Large atypical astrocytes, Alzheimer type I astrocytes, are commonly

encountered in the setting of progressive multifocal leukoencephalopathy.

92. D (Chapter 3.X.C)   The collection of epithelioid histocytes represents a non-necrotizing granuloma.

93. B (Chapter 3.X.C)   Granulomas may be seen in germinomas. The large cells seen here represent malignant germ cells.

94. C (Chapter 3.X.C)   Germinomas are most likely to arise in young males in the pineal gland region.

95. B (Chapter 2.IV.D)   The sinusoidal-type vessels arranged in a back-to-back fashion is characteristic of a cavernous angioma.

96. E (Chapter 3.VIII.B)   The elongated "tennis-racket"-like structures seen here represent Birbeck granules.

97. D (Chapter 3.VIII.B)   Birbeck granules are a distinctive feature of Langerhans cell histiocytes of histiocytosis X.

98. D (Chapter 3.VIII.B)   Langerhan's cell histiocytes stain with CD1a antibody.

99. B (Chapter 9.V.D)   The lesion seen here represents cysticercosis.

100. A (Chapter 9.V.D)   The organism responsible for cysticerosis is *Taenia solium* (the pork tapeworm).

101. D (Chapter 3.I.D)   The mildly increased cellularity and larger cells with abundant eosinophilic cytoplasm are characteristic of reactive astrocytosis.

102. B (Chapter 3.I.F)   The lesion denoted here represents glomeruloid vascular proliferation.

103. D (Chapter 3.I.A)   The prominent vascular proliferation in this astrocytoma is sufficient enough to warrant a diagnosis of WHO grade IV astrocytoma.

104. D (Chapter 1.I.H)   The loose arrangement of spindled cells is characteristic of the pituitary neurohypophysis.

105. A (Chapter 1.I.H)   The area seen here may represent either the caudate or putamen.

106. C (Chapter 1.I.H)   The fascicles of myelinated fibers seen in the caudate are known as the pencil bundles of Wilson.

107. A (Chapter 1.I.H)   The presence of the external granular cell layer of the cerebellum is a finding most consistent with an age of 3 mo.

108. B (Chapter 1.I.H)   The photomicrograph represents white matter parenchyma.

109. A (Chapter 2.IV.B)   The presence of arterial and venous vessels with intervening neural parenchyma is characteristic of an arteriovenous angioma.

110. B (Chapter 1.I.A)   Melanin-pigmented neurons are seen in substantia nigra, locus ceruleus, and the dorsal motor nucleus of the vagus nerve.

111. E (Chapter 1.I.H)   The nests of epithelioid cells separated by fibrovascular septae is characteristic of the pituitary adenohypophysis.

112. C (Chapter 9.II.D)   The central necrosis rimmed by a collagenous wall is characteristic of an organizing abscess.

113. B (Chapter 9.V.C)   The granules of darkly pigmented material within red cells in blood vessel lumina is characteristic of malaria.

114. A (Chapter 9.IV.L)   The organisms seen here have the characteristic ultrastructural appearance of cytomegalovirus.

115. E (Chapter 9.IV.L)   In an immunocompromised adult, cytomegalovirus infection most commonly manifests as microglial nodules.

116. C (Chapter 6.I.D)   Neutrophils are not a salient feature microscopically of multiple sclerosis.

117. D (Chapter 2.II.C,D)   Cavitary changes in the cortex with surrounding gliosis and a relative sparing of the molecular layer is consistent with a remote infarct.

118. E (Chapter 2.II.C,D)   Remote infarct findings are seen in association with the 3 mo of age parameter.

119. A (Chapter 1.I.A)   The cell shown here represents a neuron.

120. B (Chapter 1.I.A)   Cytoplasmic swelling with loss and peripheralization of Nissl substance and eccentric nucleus are salient features of central chromatolysis.

121. E (Chapter 1.I.H)   The section is from the cerebellum with the molecular layer to the left, and two large Purkinje cells and smaller round granular cells to the right.

122. A (Chapter 1.I.A)   The Purkinje cells are marked by ischemic changes—shrunken cell bodies with dark-staining nuclei and indistinguishable nucleoli.

123. B (Chapter 7.I.B)   The accumulation of GM2 ganglioside material is a feature of Tay-Sachs disease.

124. D (Chapter 7.I.B) The distended cells represented neurons filled with GM2 ganglioside material.

125. C (Chapter 8.IV.C) Lewy bodies are often encountered in substantia nigra (neuromelanin-pigmented) neurons.

126. D (Chapter 1.I.B) The proliferation of cells in the region of the Purkinje cell layer are the Bergmann astrocytes.

127. D (Chapter 1.I.B) Loss of Purkinje cells with astrocytosis is associated with all of the listed conditions except infiltrating astrocytoma.

128. C (Chapter 9.IV.G) The antecedent measles infection with Cowdry A inclusions is typical of SSPE (subacute sclerosing panencephalitis)

129. C (Chapter 3.IV.B) This meningioma is brain invasive, a feature some associate with malignancy.

130. C (Chapter 6.II.B) Collections of white matter globoid cells is characteristic of Krabbe's disease or globoid cell leukodystrophy.

131. B (Chapter 6.II.B) Krabbe's disease is the result of a deficiency in galactocerebroside-B galactosidase.

132. C (Chapter 6.II.B) Krabbe's disease is inherited as an autosomal recessive condition.

133. B (Chapter 7.II.B) The bilateral basal ganglia hemorrhagic necrosis is a feature of methanol toxicity.

134. C (Chapter 2.III.A) The lesion denoted by the arrow represents a saccular aneurysm arising from the posterior inferior cerebellar artery (PICA).

135. D (Chapter 2.III.A) Loss of the media defines the saccular aneurysm.

136. A (Chapter 2.III.C) There is evidence of friable, necrotic tissue consistent with infarct involving the cerebellum.

137. A (Chapter 2.IV.C) The lesion shown here represents part of a vascular malformation (venous angioma).

138. E (Chapter 1.I.B) The nuclear swelling and chromatin clearing is characteristic of an Alzheimer type II astrocyte.

139. D (Chapter 1.I.B) Alzheimer type II astrocytes are most likely encountered in hepatic encephalopathy (elevated ammonia levels).

140. C (Chapter 5.II.O) The changes seen are characteristic of bilirubin encephalopathy (kernicterus).

141. B (Chapter 4.I.B) The changes seen (expansion of gyri and narrowing of sulci) are characteristic of cerebral edema.

142. C (Chapter 2.II.C) The cavitary defect represents a remote infarct.

143. C (Chapter 4.II.B) The hemorrhage seen here represents a subdural hematoma.

144. B (Chapter 4.II.B) Subdural hematomas are associated with tearing of bridging veins which transverse through the subarachnoid space.

145. D (Chapter 2.VII.B) The thickened vessel walls with granularity is highly suggestive of CADASIL.

146. C (Chapter 2.VII.B) The notch 3 gene responsible for CADASIL is located on chromosome 19q12.

147. C (Chapter 2.II.D) The lesion seen here represents an acute infarct surrounded by a zone of edema in a pseudolaminar configuration (involving more than one cortical layer).

148. C (Chapter 2.II.D) The asymetrical loss of corticospinal tracts is likely related to an ipsilateral cerebral infarct.

149. C (Chapter 2.VI.A) The changes seen are those of a granulomatous vasculitis.

150. D (Chapter 10.III.G) The organisms seen in the skeletal muscle represents Sarcocystis infection.

151. E (Chapter 9.V.G) The elongated organism represents Strongyloides in a patient who had disseminated disease.

152. A (Chapter 9.II.F) The collection of epithelioid histiocytes and lymphocytes represents a granuloma.

153. B (Chapter 9.II.F) The best combination of stains to further evaluate this lesion would be a GMS (for fungal organisms) and fite stain (for a mycobacterial organism).

154. A (Chapter 9.II.C) Listeria infection typically presents with a suppurative leptomeningitis with abscess formation, usually not accompanied by granulomas. All of the other conditions may be associated with granuloma formation.

155. B (Chapter 4.I.D) The midline brain stem hemorrhage represents a Duret hemorrhage.

156. A (Chapter 4.I.D) The Duret hemorrhage is typically associated with uncal or lateral transtentorial herniation.

157. B (Chapter 5.I.C) The disorganized cortical architecture is a common pattern of cortical dysplasia.

158. B (Chapter 5.III.C)   The enlarged gyrus represents a cortical tuber.

159. D (Chapter 7.I.T)   The findings seen here are most consistent with those of subacute combined degeneration due to vitamin B_{12} deficiency.

160. E (Chapter 7.I.S)   Discoloration in the mamillary bodies with gliosis due to hemorrhage/hemosiderin and loss of neurons is seen in the setting of Wernicke encephalopathy.

161. C (Chapter 7.I.S)   Thiamine deficiency underlies the pathologic changes seen with Wernicke encephalopathy.

162. A (Chapter 5.I.J)   Focal neuronal loss and gliosis in the hippocampus (especially CA1, CA4, and dentate regions) characterizes hippocampal sclerosis.

163. C (Chapter 9.II.C)   The leptomeningeal vessel shows evidence of vasculitis and organizing thrombus.

164. B (Chapter 1.I.B)   The GFAP immunostain is highlighting astrocytic cells in the cortex.

165. B (Chapter 7.II.C)   The cerebellar vermal atrophy seen here is most likely related to ethanol.

166. B (Chapter 2.II.C)   The areas of darker discoloration represent multifocal acute infarcts, most likely embolic in origin.

167. C (Chapter 1.II.I)   The lesion denoted by the arrow represents a muscle spindle (intrafusal fibers enclosed by a connective tissue capsule).

168. A (Chapter 10.IV.B and Chapter 8.IV.N)   The rounded myofiber atrophy in this infant is characteristic of Werdnig-Hoffman disease.

169. B (Chapter 10.IV.B and Chapter 8.IV.N)   There is often sparing of Onuf's nucleus in Werdnig-Hoffman disease.

170. A (Chapter 10.III.I)   The changes seen in the vessel are those of a necrotizing vasculitis (polyarteritis nodosa).

171. A (Chapter 10.III.A)   Chronic endomysial inflammation in the absence of perifascicular atrophy is consistent with polymyositis.

172. A (Chapter 10.III.B)   The perifascicular pattern of injury is consistent with dermatomyositis.

173. C (Chapter 10.III.B)   Dermatomyositis is usually responsive to steroid therapy.

174. C (Chapter 10.III.C)   The vacuoles seen represent rimmed vacuoles or autophagic vacuoles.

175. D (Chapter 10.III.C)   Rimmed vacuoles in the setting of an inflammatory myopathy are highly suggestive of inclusion body myositis.

176. A (Chapter 10.VIII.F)   Ring fibers are marked by a ring of myofibrils that is oriented circumferentially around the longitudinally oriented fibrils in the rest of the fiber.

177. C (Chapter 10.VIII.F)   Ring fibers are a relatively common finding in patients with myotonic dystrophy.

178. A (Chapter 10.I.D)   The dark fibers are type I on ATPase pH 4.6.

179. B (Chapter 10.I.D)   Regenerating myofibers are highlighted on the alkaline phosphatase stain.

180. B (Chapter 10.III.C)   The tubulofilaments seen within this myofiber nucleus are characteristic of those seen in inclusion body myositis.

181. E (Chapter 1.II.G)   The dark band marked by the arrow represents the Z band.

182. E (Chapter 10.I.C)   The holes seen in all of the myofibers represent a freeze artifact sustained during processing of the biopsy specimen.

183. B (Chapter 10.VI.A)   The paracrystalline inclusions are observed in mitochondria.

184. B (Chapter 10.VI.A)   Ragged red fibers is a light microscopic finding also associated with mitochondrial myopathies.

185. D (Chapter 10.I.D)   The partial cytochrome oxidase deficiency may be indicative of a mitochondrial abnormality.

186. B (Chapter 7.I.F)   Ultrastructural evidence of curvilinear bodies supports a diagnosis of ceroid lipofucinosis.

187. D (Chapter 1.III.F)   The cystalloid structures within the Schwann cell cytoplasm are pi granules of Reich.

188. C (Chapter 1.III.E)   The structure denoted by the larger arrow is an unmyelinated axon.

189. C (Chapter 11.III.I)   The congophilic material represents amyloid deposition.

190. C (Chapter 11.III.I)   Mutations in the transthyretin or prealbumin gene are associated with hereditary forms of amyloid neuropathy.

191. A (Chapter 1.III.F)   The cell nucleus is from a Schwann cell.

192. D (Chapter 11.III.F)   The onion bulb structure is most commonly associated with Charcot-Marie-Tooth disease.

193. A (Chapter 11.III.I)   The fragmentation of myelin is consistent with axonal degeneration, a prominent feature of vasculitic neuropathy.

194. A (Chapter 11.II.A)   The changes here are consistent with axonal regeneration (sprouting).

195. C (Chapter 10.VIII.C)   The marked variation in fiber size and fibrosis are most suggestive of a dystrophic process. The clinical history favors Duchenne muscular dystrophy.

196. D (Chapter 10.VIII.C)   Dystrophin analysis would be most useful in confirming the diagnosis of Duchenne muscular dystrophy.

197. D (Chapter 10.IV.A)   The three zones of staining (central pale, dark intermediate, and normal peripheral) is characteristic of target fibers.

198. D (Chapter 10.IV.A)   Target fibers are a common feature of neurogenic atrophy.

199. B (Chapter 1.II.D)   Fascicular atrophy is associated with spinal muscular atrophy.

200. C (Chapter 10.VI.B)   The lysosomal associated (acid phosphatase positive) acid maltase deficiency is associated with glycogen (PAS positive) accumulation in vacuoles.

14 Written Self-Assessment Questions

1. Nissl substance is composed of

   A. Smooth endoplasmic reticulum

   B. Rough endoplasmic reticulum

   C. Golgi structures

   D. Neuromelanin

   E. Lipofuscin

2. Anoxic damage related to carbon monoxide poisoning would be best classified as

   A. Anoxic anoxia

   B. Anemic anoxia

   C. Histotoxic anoxia

   D. Stagnant anoxia

   E. None of the above

3. What WHO grade is pleomorphic xanthoastrocytoma?

   A. Grade I

   B. Grade II

   C. Grade III

   D. Grde IV

   E. Does not have WHO grade

4. Cerebral edema is marked by all of the following except

   A. Increased brain weight

   B. Narrowing of sulci

   C. Decreased ventricular size

   D. Narrowing of gyri

   E. Prominent pacchionian granulations

5. Meckel-Gruber syndrome is associated with all of the following except

   A. Autosomal dominant pattern of inheritance

   B. Occipital encephalocele

   C. Polydactyly

   D. Polycystic kidneys

   E. Hepatic fibrosis

6. Which HLA type is associated with the development of multiple sclerosis?

   A. HLA B7

   B. HLA D8

   C. HLA DR15

   D. HLA DW6

   E. HLA DR4

7. All of the following are "normal" aging changes in the brain except

   A. Loss of brain weight

   B. Leptomeningeal thickening

   C. Increased corpora amylacea

   D. Rare neurofibrillary tangles

   E. Decreased astrocyte number and size

8. The most common organism responsible for an intracranial epidural abscess is

   A. *E. coli*

   B. Staphylococcus

   C. Streptococcus

   D. Listeria

   E. Gram-negative anaerobes

9. The alkaline phosphatase stain is useful for identifying
   - A. Degenerating myofibers
   - B. Regenerating myofibers
   - C. Acutely denervated fibers
   - D. Mitochondrial abnormalities
   - E. Amyloid deposition

10. Congenital dilatation of the central canal is known as
    - A. Syrinx
    - B. Syringobulbia
    - C. Hydromyelia
    - D. Diplomyelia
    - E. Myeloschisis

11. Histologically, all of the following are features of multiple sclerosis except
    - A. Neutrophils
    - B. Lymphocytes
    - C. Reactive astrocytes
    - D. Macrophages
    - E. Myelin loss

12. All of the following features are characteristic of neurogenic muscle disease except
    - A. Angular atrophic fibers
    - B. Target fibers
    - C. Group atrophy
    - D. Fiber type grouping
    - E. Ring fibers

13. Marinesco bodies are most likely going to be found in which cell type?
    - A. Neuron
    - B. Astrocyte
    - C. Oligodendrocyte
    - D. Ependymal cell
    - E. Arachnoidal cap cell

14. The most senstive neurons to anoxic damage are in what region?
    - A. Endplate of hippocampus
    - B. Sommer sector
    - C. Cortex layer IV
    - D. Thalamus
    - E. Pons

15. The most common site of origin for low-grade fibrillary astrocytoma is
    - A. Frontal lobe
    - B. Parietal lobe
    - C. Temporal lobe
    - D. Occipital lobe
    - E. Spinal cord

16. Cerebral edema as a result of an impaired cell Na-K membrane pump is referred to as
    - A. Vasogenic
    - B. Cytotoxic
    - C. Tumoral
    - D. Transient
    - E. None of the above

17. Area cerebrovasculosa is associated with
    - A. Anencephaly
    - B. Meningocele
    - C. Chiari malformation
    - D. Edwards syndrome
    - E. Schizencephaly

18. Acute-onset multiple sclerosis with prominent optic nerve and spinal cord involvement represents which subtype?
    - A. Marburg type
    - B. Baló type
    - C. Schilder type
    - D. Dévic type
    - E. Concentric sclerosis type

19. Phosphorylated tau protein is associated with the development of
    - A. Neurofibrillary tangles
    - B. Neuritic plaques
    - C. Amyloid angiopathy
    - D. Granulovacuolar degeneration
    - E. Hirano bodies

20. All of the following are potential complications of bacterial leptomeningitis except
    - A. Infarct
    - B. Hemorrhage
    - C. Demyelination
    - D. Vasculitis
    - E. Hydrocephalus

21. Which of the following is the most likely cause of meningitis in a 2-wk-old infant?

    A. *Staph. epidermidis*

    B. *Staph. aureus*

    C. *Strep. agalactiae*

    D. *Strep. pneumoniae*

    E. *Listeria*

22. Cyclopia is most commonly associated with

    A. Down's syndrome

    B. Holoprosencephaly

    C. Chiari malformation, type II

    D. Dandy-Walker syndrome

    E. None of the above

23. Myofibers with basophilic cytoplasm, nuclear enlargement, and prominent nucleation are characteristic of

    A. Targetoid fibers

    B. Degenerating fibers

    C. Regenerating fibers

    D. Nemaline rods

    E. Moth-eaten fibers

24. All are characteristic of an axonal degenerative process except

    A. Axonal sprouting

    B. Myelin ovoids

    C. Bands of Bungner

    D. Macrophages

    E. Shortened internodal distances

25. Bergmann astrocytes are found in the

    A. Basal ganglia

    B. Cerebral cortex

    C. Subcortical white matter

    D. Cerebellum

    E. Hippocampus

26. Hypoglycemic neuronal necrosis preferentially affects all of the following areas except

    A. Cortex—layers II and III

    B. CA1 region of hippocampus

    C. Dentate

    D. Caudate

    E. Purkinje cells

27. All of the following are features of gliosis as opposed to diffuse astrocytoma except

    A. Rosenthal fibers

    B. Collagen deposition

    C. Microcystic change

    D. Absent calcification

    E. Reactive astrocytes

28. Kernohan's notch is associated with which of the following?

    A. Central herniation

    B. Subfalcial herniation

    C. Uncal herniation

    D. Tonsillar herniation

    E. Upward herniation

29. All of the following are commonly associated with the Chiari type I malformation except

    A. Cerebellar tonsillar herniation

    B. Adult presentation

    C. Syringomyelia

    D. Klippel-Feil anomaly

    E. Arachnoidal adhesions

30. Waterhouse-Friderichsen syndrome is most typically associated with which organism?

    A. Group B Strep

    B. *E. coli*

    C. *Listeria*

    D. *N. meningitidis*

    E. *H. influenza*

31. All of the following conditions are associated with granulomatous inflammation in the CNS except

    A. Tuberculosis

    B. Listeriosis

    C. Sarcoidosis

    D. Foreign body giant-cell reaction

    E. Coccidioidomycosis

32. All of the following are features of acute hemorrhagic leukoencephalitis except

    A. Cerebral edema

    B. Vessel wall necrosis

    C. White matter hemorrhages

    D. Immunocompromised state

    E. About half of cases present with antecedent upper respiratory infection

33. Neurofibrillary cytoskeletal alterations are a feature of which toxicity?

    A. Carbon monoxide

    B. Aluminum

    C. Arsenic

    D. Lead

    E. Manganese

34. β-Amyloid is encoded for on chromosome

    A. 1

    B. 14

    C. 19

    D. 21

    E. 22

35. All of the following are features of polymyositis except

    A. May be associated with rheumatoid arthritis

    B. CPK often elevated

    C. Endomysial chronic inflammation

    D. Autophagic vacuoles

    E. More common in females

36. The most distinguishing feature pathologically of dermatomyositis is

    A. Chronic inflammation

    B. Myofiber degeneration

    C. Myofiber regeneration

    D. Perifascicular atrophy

    E. Fascicular atrophy

37. Rosenthal fibers may be encountered in all of the following conditions except

    A. Alexander's disease

    B. Reactive astrocytosis

    C. Fibrillary astrocytoma

    D. Pilocytic astrocytoma

    E. Pineal gland cyst

38. Cerebral blood flow constitutes approximately what percentage of cardiac output?

    A. 5%

    B. 10%

    C. 15%

    D. 20%

    E. 30%

39. All of the following are genetic alterations associated with diffuse astrocytoma except

    A. *p53* mutations

    B. Increased PDGFR alpha expression

    C. Gain 7q

    D. Trisomy 22

    E. Loss of heterozygosity 10p

40. Which vessel may get compressed in lateral transtentorial herniation resulting in infarct of the calcarine cortex?

    A. Basilar artery

    B. Posterior cerebral

    C. Posterior inferior cerebellar artery

    D. Anterior inferior cerebellar artery

    E. None of the above

41. Hypoplasia of the cerebellar vermis with cystic dilatation of the 4th ventricle and agenesis of the corpus callosum would be most accurately termed

    A. Chiari type II malformation

    B. Dandy-Walker syndrome

    C. Cerebellar dysplasia

    D. Holotelencephaly

    E. Schizencephaly

42. Which of the following stains is most useful in highlighting mycobacterial organisms?

    A. Hematoxylin and eosin

    B. PAS

    C. GMS

    D. Ziehl-Neelsen

    E. Dieterle

43. Which of the following is true regarding metachromatic leukodystrophy?

    A. Chromosome 21q gene defect

    B. Autosomal dominant

    C. Arcuate U fibers not spared

    D. White matter with macrophages filled with glucocerebrosides

    E. Arylsulfatase A deficiency

44. CERAD criteria for the diagnosis of Alzheimer's disease rely on which pathologic feature?

    A. Neurofibrillary tangles

    B. Neuritic plaques

    C. Amyloid angiopathy

    D. Lewy bodies

    E. None of the above

45. All are features of dermatomyositis except
    A. Steroid refractory
    B. Heliotropic rash
    C. Gottron's papules
    D. Soft tissue calcinosis
    E. Association with malignancy

46. Miller-Dieker syndrome is associated with agyria related to deletion on chromosome 17 involving which gene?
    A. LIS-1
    B. *p53*
    C. N-*myc*
    D. Retinoblastoma gene
    E. None of the above

47. All of the following are common features of meningovascular syphilitic CNS infection except
    A. Prominent plasma cell infiltrates
    B. Gummata
    C. Heubner's endarteritis obliterans
    D. Arteritis
    E. Demyelination

48. All are true regarding or seen with inclusion body myositis except
    A. Steroid resistent
    B. Caused by viral infection
    C. Rimmed vacuoles
    D. Tubulofilamentous inclusions ultrastructurally
    E. Mitochondrial abnormalities

49. Alzheimer's II astrocytes are most commonly associated with what condition?
    A. Hepatic encephalopathy
    B. Progressive multifocal leukoencephalopathy
    C. Gliosis
    D. Pilocytic astrocytoma
    E. Alexander's disease

50. Macrophages may be first microscopically evident in an infarct at what time?
    A. Within 12 h
    B. 24 h
    C. 48 h
    D. 1 wk
    E. 3–4 wk

51. The most common glioma type in the CNS is
    A. Oligodendroglioma
    B. Ependymoma
    C. Glioblastoma multiforme
    D. Low-grade diffuse astrocytoma
    E. Pilocytic astrocytoma

52. Rupture of the middle meningeal artery is associated with
    A. Duret hemorrhage
    B. Epidural hemorrhage
    C. Subdural hemorrhage
    D. Subarachnoid hemorrhage
    E. Parenchymal hemorrhage

53. Cortical dysplasia is associated with all of the following except
    A. Tuberous sclerosis
    B. Dysembryoplastic neuroepithelial tumor
    C. Neurofibromatosis type I
    D. Neurofibromatosis type II
    E. Epidermal nevus syndrome

54. All are true regarding globoid cell leukodystrophy except
    A. Deficiency of galactocerebrosidase
    B. Autosomal recessive
    C. Onset of symptoms in first year of life
    D. Sparing of arcuate subcortical fibers
    E. Atrophy of brain

55. All of the following are pathologic features of Alzheimer's disease except
    A. Granulovacuolar degeneration
    B. Hirano bodies
    C. Bunina bodies
    D. Lewy bodies
    E. Amyloid angiopathy

56. Which fungus is a budding yeast with a thick mucopolysaccharide wall?
    A. Cryptococcus
    B. Candida
    C. Aspergillus
    D. Mucormycosis
    E. Coccidioidomycosis

57. The diabetic patient with a periorbital infection involving organisms with nonseptate hyphae is most likely infected with

    A. Aspergillus

    B. Candida

    C. Mucormycosis

    D. Blastomycosis

    E. Actinomyces

58. Lissencephaly results from defects in development that occur during the

    A. 5th–7th wk of gestation

    B. 8th–10th wk of gestation

    C. 11th–13th wk of gestation

    D. 15th–17th wk of gestation

    E. 20th–22nd wk of gestation

59. A protoplasmic body is a salient feature of which of the following?

    A. Alzheimer's disease

    B. Demyelinating disease

    C. Fungal infection

    D. Congenital myopathy

    E. Tumor

60. An infarct of what minimum volume of brain tissue will almost invariably result in dementia

    A. 10 mL

    B. 25 mL

    C. 50 mL

    D. 80 mL

    E. 120 mL

61. The "fried egg" appearance of oligodendrocytes represents

    A. Cell cytoplasm

    B. Perinuclear edema

    C. Artifact of delayed fixation

    D. Increased cytoplasmic lipid

    E. None of the above

62. The least common site for a lacunar infarct is the

    A. Putamen

    B. Caudate

    C. Pons

    D. Mamillary bodies

    E. Thalamus

63. All are features of metastatic carcinoma except

    A. Discrete gross lesion

    B. Collagenous stroma

    C. Discrete cell borders

    D. Cytokeratin immunoreactivity

    E. Perinecrotic pseudopalisading

64. An acute subdural hematoma is associated with a skull fracture (in)

    A. Never

    B. 25% of cases

    C. 50% of cases

    D. 75% of cases

    E. Almost always

65. Agyria with hydrocephalus, retinal dysplasia, encephalocele, no muscle disease, and death in infancy is most characteristic of

    A. Cerebro-ocular dysplasia

    B. Neu-Laxova syndrome

    C. Zellweger's syndrome

    D. Miller-Dieker syndrome

    E. Walker-Warburg syndrome

66. Most forms of adrenoleukodystrophy are related to an abnormality on which chromosome?

    A. 1

    B. 22

    C. 19

    D. 6

    E. None of the above

67. Target fibers are most closely associated with which process?

    A. Polymyositis

    B. Dermatomyositis

    C. Myotonic dystrophy

    D. Neurogenic atrophy

    E. Mitochondrial myopathy

68. Diphtheritic neuropathy is best classified as being

    A. The result of Schwann cell dysfunction

    B. The result of myelin sheath damage

    C. The result of vessel damage

    D. The result of axonal damage

    E. None of the above

69. Neurofibrillary tangles are best highlighted on which stain?

    A. PAS

    B. Trichrome

    C. Cytochrome oxidase

    D. Bodian

    E. Congo red

70. The Huntington gene is located on which chromosome?

    A. 1

    B. 4

    C. 14

    D. 19

    E. 21

71. Infection with which organism is associated with sulfur granule formation?

    A. Coccidioidomycosis

    B. Blastomycosis

    C. Actinomycosis

    D. Nocardiosis

    E. None of the above

72. Cowdry type A inclusions are typical of all the following organisms except

    A. Polio virus

    B. CMV

    C. Epstein-Barr virus

    D. Herpes virus

    E. JC virus

73. Ciliary body attachments in ependymal cells are known as

    A. Kinetoplasts

    B. Chloroplasts

    C. Microtubuloblasts

    D. Blepharoplasts

    E. None of the above

74. What percentage of saccular aneurysms are bilateral?

    A. < 5%

    B. 10%

    C. 20%

    D. 50%

    E. 85%

75. Eosinophilic granular bodies are a common feature of

    A. Glioblastoma multiforme

    B. Pilocytic astrocytoma

    C. Subependymal giant-cell astrocytoma

    D. Nasal glioma

    E. None of the above

76. Traumatic basilar subarachnoid hemorrhage is related to the tear of what vessel?

    A. Basilar artery

    B. Vertebral artery

    C. Subclavian artery

    D. Aorta

    E. External carotid artery

77. A brain weight of 2350 g is properly termed

    A. Megalocephaly

    B. Schizencephaly

    C. Microencephaly

    D. Megaloencephaly

    E. Normal

78. Other organ systems that frequently contain inclusions in adenoleukodystrophy include all of the following except

    A. Testis

    B. Peripheral nerve

    C. Liver

    D. Lymph nodes

    E. Pancreas

79. All of the following pathologies are typical of a CNS viral infection except

    A. Granulomas

    B. Microglial nodules

    C. Neuronophagia

    D. Chronic inflammation

    E. Central chromatolysis

80. All of the following are true regarding subacute sclerosing panencephalitis (SSPE) except

    A. Most present <15 yr of age

    B. Most recover without serious sequelae

    C. The result of measles virus infection

    D. Causes demyelination

    E. Associated with neurofibrillary tangle formation

81. Fascicular muscle atrophy is most commonly associated with

    A. Myasthenia gravis

    B. Kugelberg-Welander disease

    C. Amyotrophic lateral sclerosis

    D. Polymyositis

    E. Mitochondrial myopathy

82. Which of the following is a trinucleotide repeat disorder?

    A. Progressive supranuclear palsy

    B. Diffuse Lewy body disease

    C. Corticobasal degeneration

    D. Hallervorden-Spatz disease

    E. Huntington's chorea

83. The most common site of a Morton's neuroma is the

    A. Median nerve

    B. Peroneal nerve

    C. Radial nerve

    D. Intermetatarsal nerves

    E. Sural nerve

84. All are true regarding Negri bodies except

    A. Seen in Rabies

    B. Intraneuronal

    C. Intranuclear

    D. Eosinophilic

    E. Hippocamal neurons frequently involved

85. Which of the following immunostains is a useful marker for microglial cells?

    A. GFAP

    B. Synaptophysin

    C. HAM56

    D. S-100 protein

    E. CLA

86. All of the following are conditions associated with saccular aneurysms except

    A. Tuberous sclerosis

    B. Polycystic kidney disease

    C. Coarctation of the aorta

    D. Marfan's syndrome

    E. Ehler-Danlos syndrome

87. All are features of the pleomorphic xanthoastrocytoma except

    A. Temporal lobe location

    B. Cyst with enhancing mural nodule radiographically

    C. Reticulin rich

    D. Nuclear pleomorphism

    E. Increased mitotic activity

88. Langerhans cell histocytosis is characteristically marked by which antibody?

    A. CD1a

    B. CD1b

    C. CD1c

    D. CD4

    E. CD8

89. "Raccoon eyes" are associated with

    A. Hinge fracture

    B. Basilar skull fracture

    C. Diastatic fracture

    D. Frontal depressed skull fracture

    E. None of the above

90. All of the following are characteristic of Down's syndrome except

    A. Reduced frontal lobe

    B. Narrowing of the inferior temporal gyrus

    C. Small cerebellum

    D. Poor myelination

    E. Alzheimer-like pathology in middle-aged adults

91. Which of the following is a characteristic feature of Alexander's disease?

    A. Megalencephaly

    B. Arcuate subcortical fibers spared

    C. Eosinophilic granular bodies

    D. Presents typically in the 2nd decade of life

    E. Phospholipid protein defect

92. A grossly normal brain with gliosis in the caudate and putamen translates into what Vonsattel grade for Huntington's chorea?

    A. Grade 0

    B. Grade 1

    C. Grade 2

    D. Grade 3

    E. Grade 4

93. The spread of which organism from the periphery to the central nervous system occurs primarily via retrograde axoplasmic transport?

    A. Poliovirus

    B. Arbovirus

    C. CMV

    D. Herpes virus

    E. PML

94. Hippocampal sclerosis is characterized by marked loss of neurons in which location?

    A. Caudate

    B. Amygdala

    C. Sommer sector

    D. CA2

    E. None of the above

95. Circulating antibodies to the acetylcholine receptor are seen in

    A. McArdle's disease

    B. MELAS syndrome

    C. Myasthenia gravis

    D. Lambert-Eaton syndrome

    E. None of the above

96. All are true regarding Guillian-Barre syndrome except

    A. Associated with HLA B27

    B. Ascending paralysis

    C. Decreased deep tendon reflexes

    D. Endoneurial chronic inflammation

    E. Segmental demyelination

97. Layer III of the cerebral cortex is known as the

    A. External granular layer

    B. Internal granular layer

    C. Polymorphic layer

    D. Outer pyramidal layer

    E. Inner pyramidal layer

98. Dolichoectasia is associated with the development of which of the following?

    A. Fusiform aneurysm

    B. Mycotic aneurysm

    C. Saccular aneurysm

    D. Berry aneurysm

    E. Charcot aneurysm

99. All of the following are true regarding ganglio-glioma except

    A. Most commonly arise in temporal lobe

    B. Associated with cortical dysplasia

    C. Associated with chronic epilepsy

    D. Frequently contain small necrotic foci that do not alter its good prognosis

    E. Calcifications common

100. A zellballen architectural pattern microscopically characterizes which tumor?

    A. Schwannoma

    B. Neurofibroma

    C. Ependymoma

    D. Paraganglioma

    E. Chordoma

101. The wounding capacity of a gunshot wound is most related to

    A. Size of bullet

    B. Shape of bullet

    C. Velocity of bullet

    D. Weight of bullet

    E. Size of gun

102. Focal coagulative necrosis adjacent to the lateral ventricles in a 30-wk-old fetus is best termed

    A. Ulegyria

    B. Multilocular cystic encephalomalacia

    C. Periventricular leukomalacia

    D. Diffuse lobar sclerosis

    E. Multiple sclerosis

103. Congenital CMV infection is characterized by all the following except

    A. Chorioretinitis

    B. Gliosis

    C. Hydrocephalus

    D. Megalencephaly

    E. Microcephaly

104. All of the following characterize Lambert-Eaton syndrome except

    A. Proximal muscle weakness

    B. Decreased neurotransmission with repeated stimulation

    C. Autonomic dysfunction

    D. Associated with small cell carcinoma of lung

    E. Antibodies to presynaptic calcium channels

105. The "motor oil" appearance of fluid in a cystic craniopharyngioma is the result of

    A. Cholesterol

    B. Keratin

    C. Necrosis

    D. Calcification

    E. Glycogen

106. Leprosy-associated neuropathy may be marked by all of the following except

    A. Granulomas

    B. Schwann cell invasion by organisms

    C. Perineurial fibrosis

    D. Symmetric polyneuropathy

    E. Toxin-mediated response

107. Autosomal dominant transmission of Parkinson's disease is linked with what gene?

    A. Tau protein gene

    B. Agitonian

    C. Ubiquitin

    D. α-Synuclein

    E. SOD1

108. Nemaline rods are composed of

    A. α-Actinin

    B. Dystrophin

    C. Emerin

    D. Sarcoplasmic reticulum

    E. None of the above

109. The pencil bundles of Wilson are a feature of which structure?

    A. Substantia nigra

    B. Dentate

    C. Putamen

    D. Locus ceruleus

    E. Hippocampus

110. The most common organism associated with the development of mycotic aneurysms is

    A. Mucor

    B. Aspergillus

    C. Candida

    D. Cryptococcus

    E. Blastomycosis

111. Chemoresponsiveness in anaplastic oligodendrogliomas has been linked to deletions on which chromosome?

    A. 1

    B. 3

    C. 11

    D. 17

    E. 22

112. Static-loading blunt head injury is the result of forces applied gradually to the head, such as with a

    A. Car rolling over a head

    B. Hammer blow to head

    C. Gunshot to head

    D. Trauma sustained in a landslide

    E. Pedestrian hit by a car

113. All of the following are common sites of bilirubin deposition in kernicterus except

    A. Dentate

    B. Inferior olive

    C. Cranial nerve nucleus VIII

    D. Claustrum

    E. Substantia nigra

114. Canavan's disease is the result of a deficiency in

    A. Arylsulfatase B

    B. Lipophosphorylase

    C. Aspartoacylase

    D. Proteolipid protein

    E. Not known

115. All of the following are common features of the congenital myopathies except

    A. Disorders of myofiber maturation/reorganization

    B. Often fatal

    C. Retarded motor development

    D. Associated with skeletal dysmorphism

    E. Many show familial tendencies

116. All of the following are true regarding Lyme-associated neuropathy except

    A. Caused by *Borrelia burgdorferi*

    B. Acquired from a mosquito bite

    C. May be associated with arthritis

    D. Perivascular chronic inflammation

    E. Axonal degeneration

117. For those hard-to-identify Lewy bodies, which of the following stains would be most useful?

    A. PAS

    B. Congo red

    C. Ubiquitin

    D. GFAP

    E. Gomori methenamine silver

118. Which of the following is true regarding progressive multifocal leukoencephalopathy?

    A. Caused by RNA virus

    B. Most patients present <age 12 yr

    C. Alzheimer's II astrocytes

    D. Gray matter microglial nodules

    E. Oligodendroglial cell inclusions

119. Vacuolar myelopathy is a feature of

    A. Syphilis

    B. HIV

    C. HTLV-I

    D. PML

    E. None of the above

120. Ragged red fibers may be seen in all the following except

    A. MELAS

    B. MERFF

    C. Kearns-Sayre syndrome

    D. Inclusion body myositis

    E. Central core myopathy

121. The endplate of the hippocampus (Ammon's horn) is referred to as

    A. Dentate

    B. CA1

    C. CA2

    D. CA3

    E. CA4

122. Which vascular malformation is characterized by back-to-back vessels?

    A. AVM

    B. Venous angioma

    C. Cavernous angioma

    D. Capillary telangiectasia

    E. Varix

123. All are true regarding central neurocytoma except

    A. Presents usually in young adults

    B. Most patients die within 2 yr of diagnosis

    C. Synaptophysin positive

    D. Intraventricular location

    E. Dense secretory core granules ultrastructurally

124. A "burst lobe" represents an example of a

    A. Skull fracture

    B. Gunshot wound

    C. Coup contusion

    D. Contrecoup lesion

    E. Gliding contusion

125. The neurofibromin gene is located on chromosome

    A. 1

    B. 22

    C. 3

    D. 9

    E. 17

126. The salient pathologic features of Pelizaeus-Merzbacher disease include all of the following except

    A. Perivascular demyelination

    B. Brain atrophy

    C. Astrocytosis

    D. Prominent cerebellar and brain stem involvement

    E. White matter macrophages

127. Which of the following is not true regarding HTLV-I infection?

    A. Caused by retrovirus

    B. Causes tropical spastic paraparesis

    C. Myelin loss in spinal cord

    D. Cowdry A viral inclusions

    E. Demyelination of optic nerve

128. Paraneoplastic neuropathy is most commonly associated with which tumor type?

    A. Breast carcinoma

    B. Lung carcinoma

    C. Melanoma

    D. Lymphoma

    E. Renal cell carcinoma

129. Where should one look for Lewy bodies?

    A. Neuronal nucleus

    B. Neuronal cytoplasm

    C. Astrocytic nucleus

    D. Astrocytic cytoplasm

    E. Both neuronal and astrocytic cytoplasm

130. All of the following may be seen with Kearns-Sayre syndrome except

    A. Deafness

    B. Acromegaly

    C. Ophthalmoplegia

    D. Retinitis pigmentosa

    E. Heart block

131. Straight filament (tau positive) tangles with gliosis and neuropil threads in the basal ganglia and brain stem region support a diagnosis of

    A. Alzheimer's disease

    B. Progressive supranuclear palsy

    C. Striatonigral degeneration

    D. Corticobasal degeneration

    E. None of the above

132. Type II glycogenosis is related to a defect on chromosome

    A. 1

    B. 12

    C. 17

    D. 22

    E. X

133. Perifascicular atrophy is a feature of

    A. Dermatomyositis

    B. Polymyositis

    C. Neurogenic atrophy

    D. Myotonic dystrophy

    E. Steroid use

134. The most common cause of nontraumatic hemorrhage is

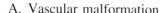

    A. Vascular malformation

    B. Aneurysm

    C. Coagulopathy

    D. Hypertension

    E. Vasculitis

135. The most important feature in predicting the outcome in ependymomas is

    A. Mitosis counts

    B. Presence of necrosis

    C. Cellularity

    D. Vascular proliferation

    E. Extent of resection

136. All of the following areas are common sites of diffuse axonal injury except the

    A. Midbrain

    B. Corpus callosum

    C. Fornix

    D. Corona radiata

    E. Superior cerebellar peduncles

137. Which of the following is a major diagnostic criterion for neurofibromatosis type I?

    A. Six or more café-au-lait spots >15 mm in a child

    B. One plexiform neurofibroma

    C. One Lisch nodule

    D. Cousin with neurofibromatosis type I.

    E. Facial freckling

138. A distinguishing feature of myxopapillary ependymoma versus ordinary ependymoma is

    A. Pseudorosettes

    B. True rosettes

    C. GFAP positivity

    D. Mucoid stroma

    E. Papillary architecture

139. The most common pathologic manifestation of Toxoplasmosis infection in the CNS in an immunocompromised adult is

    A. Abscess

    B. Hemorrhage

    C. Infarct

    D. Leptomeningitis

    E. Granulomas

140. Glycogen storage diseases are manifested typically on a muscle biopsy by

    A. Myonecrosis

    B. Vacuolar changes

    C. Extensive fibrosis

    D. Fascicular atrophy

    E. Targetoid fibers

141. Dürcks nodes are a feature of

    A. CMV

    B. Toxoplasmosis

    C. Amebiasis

    D. Malaria

    E. None of the above

142. All are true regarding Hallervorden-Spatz disease except

    A. Onset in childhood

    B. Autosomal dominant

    C. May cause choreoathetosis

    D. Globus pallidus rust brown colored

    E. Increased iron deposition in brain

143. Cysticercosis is caused by

    A. Pork tapeworm

    B. Beef tapeworm

    C. Liver fluke

    D. Lung fluke

    E. Nematode

144. Anti-MAG antibodies are most commonly associated with

    A. Paraneoplastic neuropathy

    B. Myasthenia gravis

    C. Dysproteinemic neuropathy

    D. Guillian-Barre disease

    E. None of the above

145. The longitudinal boundaries defining the sarcomere are the

    A. A bands

    B. I bands

    C. M lines

    D. Z bands

    E. H bands

146. All of the following are true regarding amyloid angiopathy except

    A. Associated with Down's syndrome

    B. Cause of lobar hemorrhage

    C. Highlighted with a congo red stain

    D. Chromosome 21 abnormality

    E. Associated with Pick's disease

147. Meningiomas with a high likelihood of recurrence include all of the following except

    A. Metaplastic

    B. Rhabdoid

    C. Papillary

    D. Clear cell

    E. Atypical

148. Neurofibromatosis type II is related to abnormality on chromosome

    A. 1

    B. 17

    C. 3

    D. 22

    E. 9

149. Tay-Sachs disease is caused by a deficiency in

    A. β-Galactosidase

    B. Arylsulfatase

    C. Hexosaminidase A

    D. Glucocerebrosidase

    E. Iduronidase

150. Which of the following is true regarding type-IV glycogenosis?

    A. Myophosphorylase deficiency

    B. Autosomal dominant condition

    C. Chromosome 17 defect

    D. Females > males

    E. Normal ischemic exercise test

151. An oil-red-O stain may be most helpful in diagnosing

    A. McArdle's disease

    B. Mitochondrial disease

    C. Carnitine deficiency

    D. Myotonic dystrophy

    E. Central core myopathy

152. Chagas disease is caused by

    A. *S. japonicum*

    B. *T. gondii*

    C. *T. brucei*

    D. *T. cruzi*

    E. *T. gambiense*

153. All are true regarding Tay-Sachs disease except

   A. GM2 gangliosidosis

   B. Cherry red spot in macula

   C. Balloon neurons

   D. May see normal brain weight

   E. Hepatosplenomegaly

154. Multisystem atrophy includes which of the following conditions?

   A. Olivopontocerebellar atrophy

   B. Hallervorden-Spatz disease

   C. Corticobasal degeneration

   D. Friedrich's ataxia

   E. Huntington's disease

155. All are salient features of Creutzfeldt-Jakob pathology except

   A. Spongiform change

   B. Microglial nodules

   C. Gliosis

   D. Neuronal loss

   E. Kuru plaques

156. Charcot-Marie-Tooth disease may be caused by defects associated with which chromosomes?

   A. 1 and 9

   B. 1 and 17

   C. 9 and 17

   D. 17 and 22

   E. X and 22

157. Increased myofiber central nuclei may be seen in all of the following except

   A. Exercise-induced hypertrophy

   B. Neurogenic atrophy

   C. Myotubular myopathy

   D. Myotonic dystrophy

   E. Charcot-Marie-Tooth disease

158. Granulomatous vasculitis is a common feature of

   A. Polyarteritis nodosa

   B. Wegener's vasculitis

   C. Lupus associated vasculitis

   D. Hypersensitivity angiitis

   E. None of the above

159. The most common cytogenetic abnormality in meningiomas involves chromosome

   A. 1

   B. 2

   C. 10

   D. 17

   E. 22

160. Retraction balls or spheroids and punctate hemorrhages are most characteristic of

   A. Contusion

   B. Infarct

   C. Diffuse axonal injury

   D. Burst lobe

   E. None of the above

161. Which of the following is associated with tuberous sclerosis?

   A. Pilocytic astrocytoma

   B. Optic nerve glioma

   C. Subependymal giant cell astrocytoma

   D. Brain stem glioma

   E. Medulloblastoma

162. Abnormal accumulation of sphingomyelin and cholesterol is a feature of

   A. Tay-Sach disease

   B. Niemann-Pick disease

   C. Gaucher's disease

   D. Batten's disease

   E. Mucolipidoses

163. The most common cause of death in Friedrich's ataxia is

   A. Brain infarct/stroke

   B. Heart disease

   C. Herniation

   D. Coagulopathy related bleed

   E. Associated neoplasm

164. All are true regarding Friedrich's ataxia except

   A. Autosomal recessive

   B. Chromosome 9q defect

   C. GAA trinucleotide repeat disorder

   D. Posterior columns spared

   E. Ganglion cell/posterior root degeneration

165. The prion protein gene is located on which chromosome?

   A. 1

   B. 17

   C. 20

   D. 22

   E. None of the above

166. Dilatation of muscle sarcoplasmic reticulum with tubular aggregates is a feature of

   A. Myasthenia gravis

   B. Myoadenylate deficiency

   C. Malignant hyperthermia

   D. Periodic paralysis

   E. None of the above

167. Which is true regarding Dejerine-Sottas disease?

   A. Autosomal dominant

   B. X-linked

   C. Presents in young adulthood

   D. Nerve enlargement

   E. Primarily axonal degenerative disease

168. Phytanoyl CoA α-hydroxylase deficiency causes

   A. Fabry's disease

   B. Refsum's disese

   C. Riley-Day syndrome

   D. Canavan's disease

   E. Metachromatic leukodystrophy

169. Intermediate filaments that link Z discs together in muscle are known as

   A. Actin

   B. Desmin

   C. Myosin

   D. Dystrophin

   E. Vimentin

170. The highest yield area to look for vasculitis on a biopsy would be

   A. Leptomeninges

   B. Cerebral cortex

   C. White matter

   D. Hippocampus

   E. Basal ganglia

171. Solitary fibrous tumor can be distinguished from meningioma by immunoreactivity to

   A. Vimentin

   B. CD34

   C. S-100 protein

   D. Cytokeratins AE1/3

   E. Actin

172. A Duret hemorrhage is located in the

   A. Frontal lobe

   B. Basal ganglia

   C. Mamillary bodies

   D. Cerebellum

   E. Pons

173. All of the following are associated with tuberous sclerosis except

   A. Schwannoma

   B. Adenoma sebaceum

   C. Angiomyolipoma

   D. Cardiac rhabdomyoma

   E. Lymphangioleiomyomatosis

174. Cherry red spots in the macula is a prominent feature of all the following except

   A. Tay-Sachs disease

   B. Niemann-Pick disease

   C. Gaucher's disease

   D. Sialodosis

   E. They are seen in all of the above

175. Type IIb muscle fiber atrophy is a feature of

   A. Alcohol myopathy

   B. Steroid myopathy

   C. Chloroquine myopathy

   D. AZT myopathy

   E. Cimetidine myopathy

176. All of the following are true regarding primary CNS lymphoma except

   A. More common in males

   B. Most are B-cell type

   C. Most are diffuse small cell type

   D. Most are parenchymal based

   E. Most are angiocentric histologically

177. von Hippel-Lindau disease is associated with all of the following except

    A. Pheochromocytoma

    B. Hemangiopericytoma

    C. Renal cell carcinoma

    D. Secondary polycythemia vera

    E. Autosomal dominant inheritance pattern

178. Spinocerebellar degeneration with sensory neuropathy as a result of chronic intestinal fat malabsorption is caused by deficiency of

    A. Vitamin A

    B. Vitamin B

    C. Thiamine

    D. Vitamin E

    E. Vintamin K

179. A SOD1 gene defect on chromsome 21 is associated with what disorder?

    A. Becker's muscular dystrophy

    B. Myotonic dystrophy

    C. Refsum's disease

    D. Amyotrophic lateral sclerosis

    E. Werdnig-Hoffman disease

180. All of the following inclusions are seen frequently in amyotrophic lateral sclerosis except

    A. Hirano bodies

    B. Bunina bodies

    C. Hyaline inclusions

    D. Basophilic inclusions

    E. Skeins

181. Which of the following cells is a normal constituent of the endoneurial compartment

    A. Lymphocytes

    B. Eosinophils

    C. Mast cells

    D. Basophils

    E. Neutrophils

182. CADASIL is associated with a mutation on the notch 3 gene located on which chromosome?

    A. 1

    B. 17

    C. 19

    D. 21

    E. 22

183. Physaliphorous cells are a feature of which tumor?

    A. Meningioma

    B. Hemangioblastoma

    C. Hemangiopericytoma

    D. Chondroma

    E. None of the above

184. All of the following are autosomal dominant disorders except

    A. Neurofibromatosis type I

    B. Neurofibromatosis type II

    C. Neurocutaneous melanosis

    D. Tuberous sclerosis

    E. Sturge-Weber disease

185. A trigeminal nevus flammeus is a marker of

    A. Epidermal nevus syndrome

    B. Cowden disease

    C. Sturge-Weber disease

    D. Gorlen syndrome

    E. Tuberous sclerosis

186. Sea blue histocytes in the bone marrow are a feature of

    A. Tay-Sachs disease

    B. Niemann-Pick disease

    C. Ceroid-lipofucinosis

    D. Cystinosis

    E. Lafora body disease

187. "Giant aneurysm" is used to denote a saccular aneurysm greater than

    A. 0.5 cm

    B. 1.0 cm

    C. 1.5 cm

    D. 2.0 cm

    E. 2.5 cm

188. The most common site of origin of choroid plexus papillomas in children is

    A. Lateral ventricle

    B. Third ventricle

    C. Fourth ventricle

    D. Brain stem

    E. Spinal cord

189. Cowden syndrome is associated with which of the following?

    A. Medulloblastoma

    B. Cerebellar gangliocytoma

    C. Melanoma

    D. Lymphoma

    E. Melanotic schwannoma

190. Which of the following is the result of a defect on chromosome 1q?

    A. Niemann-Pick disease

    B. Gaucher's disease

    C. Morquio's disease

    D. Sialodosis

    E. Mucolipidoses

191. All of the following are characteristic of Leigh's disease except

    A. Associated with mitochondrial defects

    B. Autosomal recessive

    C. Most survive to early adulthood

    D. Vascular proliferation in periventricular gray matter (brain stem)

    E. Lactic acidosis

192. Ethanol is associated with all the following except

    A. Anterior vermal atrophy

    B. Peripheral neuropathy

    C. Corpus callosum demyelination

    D. Thiamine deficiency

    E. Neurofibrillary tangles

193. Lamellated cytoplasmic structures located within the Schwann cell cytoplasm that increase with age are referred to as

    A. Corpuscles of Erzholz

    B. Lipofuscin

    C. Schmidt-Lanterman clefts

    D. Pi granules of Reich

    E. Space of Klebs

194. Moyamoya is characterized by all of the following except

    A. Amyloid deposition

    B. Peak incidence in the 1st and 4th decades

    C. Females > males

    D. May see hemorrhage

    E. Vessel occlusion with intimal fibroplasia

195. Secondary polycythemia vera is associated with

    A. Hemangiopericytoma

    B. Hemangioblastoma

    C. Meningioma

    D. Solitary fibrous tumor

    E. Choroid plexus papilloma

196. The accumulation of autofluorescent lipopigments in neurons resulting in granular, fingerprint, or curvilinear inclusions by electron microscopy is known as

    A. Gaucher's disease

    B. Batten's disease

    C. Mucopolysaccharidoses

    D. Cystinosis

    E. Fucosidosis

197. Neuronal-PAS positive deposits, skin telangiectasia, renal insufficiency, and autonomic dysfunction are features of

    A. Sialodosis

    B. Tay-Sachs disease

    C. Fucosidosis

    D. Fabry's disese

    E. Lafora body disease

198. All the following are related to gene defects on the X chromosome except

    A. Fabry's disease

    B. Duchenne dystrophy

    C. Adrenoleukodystrophy

    D. Hunter's mucopolysaccharidosis

    E. Lafora body disease

199. Loss of anterior horn cells, tongue fasciculations, and hypotonia in a 2-mo-old is most likely due to a disorder associated with what chromosome?

    A. 1

    B. 5

    C. 14

    D. 16

    E. 17

200. The ratio of myelinated to unmyelinated axons in a sural nerve biopsy would be best approximated by which of the following?

    A. 1 : 2

    B. 1 : 4

    C. 1 : 6

    D. 1 : 8

    E. 1 : 10

201. The most common cause of "aseptic" meningitis is

    A. Bacteria

    B. Virus

    C. Fungus

    D. Parasite

    E. Prion protein disease

202. All are true regarding familial insomnia syndrome except

    A. Most patients survive 10-20 years

    B. Autosomal dominant

    C. Associated autonomic dysfunction

    D. A prion-protein-associated disease

    E. Thalamic gliosis

203. The saltatory conduction pattern in the peripheral nerve is most closely related to which stucture?

    A. Node of Ranvier

    B. Periaxonal space of Klebs

    C. Neurofilaments

    D. Schmidt-Lanterman clefts

    E. Vasa vasorum

204. The major defining histopathologic feature of a saccular aneurysm is

    A. Breaks in the internal elastic membrane

    B. Absence of the media

    C. Inflammation

    D. Atherosclerotic change

    E. Intimal fibroplasia

205. Genetic alterations associated with medulloblastoma most frequently involve chromosome

    A. 1

    B. 10

    C. 17

    D. 19

    E. 20

206. The single best immunomarker for medulloblastoma is which of the following?

    A. Cytokeratin

    B. GFAP

    C. S-100

    D. Synaptophysin

    E. Chromogranin

207. Poor prognosis in medulloblastoma is associated with all of the following except

    A. Age >3 yr

    B. Metastases at presentation

    C. Subtotal resection

    D. Large cell variant

    E. Melanotic variant

208. Which of the following are true regarding primary angiitis of the CNS?

    A. ESR may be normal

    B. Most common in older adults, typically >60 yr

    C. Veins involved more than arteries

    D. Marked by prominent eosinophilia

    E. Almost always granulomatosis

209. Melanotic schwannoma is associated with which of the following

    A. Turcot syndrome

    B. Cowden disease

    C. Neurofibromatosis type I

    D. Tuberous sclerosis

    E. Carney's compex

210. The most common form of hereditary amyloidosis peripheral neuropathy is related to a mutation of which gene?

    A. κ Light chain

    B. λ Light chain

    C. β-Amyloid

    D. Transthyretin

    E. Albumin

15 Answers to the Written Self-Assessment Questions

1. B (Chapter 1.I.A) Nissl substance is composed of rough endoplasmic reticulum.

2. B (Chapter 2.I.A) Carbon monoxide poisoning represents an example of anemic anoxia (insufficient oxygen content in blood).

3. B (Chapter 3.I.A) The pleomorphic xanthoastrocytoma is a WHO grade II tumor.

4. D (Chapter 4.I.B) Cerebral edema causes expansion of the gyri.

5. A (Chapter 5.I.A) Meckel-Gruber syndrome is an autosomal recessive condition.

6. C (Chapter 6.I.D) HLA-DR15 is associated with the development of multiple sclerosis.

7. E (Chapter 7.I.) Increased astrocyte number and size are seen with "normal" aging.

8. C (Chapter 9.II.A) Streptococcus is the most common cause of an intracranial epidural abscess.

9. B (Chapter 10.I.D) Alkaline phosphatase stains regenerating myofibers black.

10. C (Chapter 5.I.A) Hydromyelia is characterized by congenital dilatation of the central canal of the spinal cord.

11. A (Chapter 6.I.D) Neutrophils are not a histologic feature of the multiple sclerosis plaque.

12. E (Chapter 10.II.D) Ring fibers are more commonly encountered in myopathic processes such as muscular dystrophy.

13. A (Chapter 1.I.A) Marinesco bodies are intranuclear neuronal inclusions.

14. B (Chapter 2.I.C) Sommer sector (CA1) neurons are the most sensitive to anoxic injury.

15. A (Chapter 3.I.B) Frontal lobe (with the most white matter) is the most common site of origin for the low-grade fibrillary astrocytoma.

16. B (Chapter 4.I.C) Cytotoxic edema is caused by impairment of the cell Na-K pump.

17. A (Chapter 5.I.A) Area cerebrovasculosa (cystic mass with vessels) is associated with anencephaly.

18. D (Chapter 6.I.D) Dévic-type multiple sclerosis is characterized by predominantly optic nerve and spinal cord involvement.

19. A (Chapter 8.III.E) Phosphorylated tau proteins are associated with the development of neurofibrillary tangles.

20. C (Chapter 9.II.C) Demyelination is not a frequent complication of bacterial meningitis.

21. C (Chapter 9.II.C) *Streptococcus agalactiae* (group B) is the most common cause of neonatal bacterial meningitis (along with *E. coli*).

22. B (Chapter 5.I.B) Cyclopia is most commonly associated with holoprosencephaly.

23. C (Chapter 10.III.A) Regenerating fibers are marked by cytoplasmic basophilia, nuclear enlargement, and nucleolation.

24. E (Chapter 11.II.A) Shortened internodal distances is a feature of remyelination.

25. D (Chapter 1.I.B). Bergmann astrocytes are found in the cerebellum near the Purkinje cells.

26. E (Chapter 2.II.I) The Purkinje cells of the cerebellum are relatively spared in hypoglycemic neuronal necrosis.

27. C (Chapter 3.I.D)   True microcystic degeneration is more commonly a feature of glioma than gliosis.

28. C (Chapter 4.I.D)   Uncal or lateral transtentorial herniation may cause a Kernohan's notch (damage to contralateral cerebral peduncle).

29. D (Chapter 5.I.B)   Klippel-Feil abnormalities are more typically a feature of Chiari type II malformation.

30. D (Chapter 9.II.C)   Waterhouse-Friderichsen (adrenal gland hemorrhage) is most commonly associated with Neisseria meningitidis.

31. B (Chapter 9.II.A) Listeriosis does not usually result in granuloma formation—it more typically manifests as acute leptomeningitis with abscesses.

32. D (Chapter 6.I.F)   There is no predisposition of immunocompromised individuals to develop acute hemorrhagic leukoencephalitis.

33. B (Chapter 7.II.D)   Aluminum toxicity is associated with neurofibrillary cytoskeletal alterations.

34. D (Chapter 8.III.I)   β-Amyloid in Alzheimer's disease is encoded for on chromosome 21.

35. D (Chapter 10.III.A)   Autophagic (rimmed) vacuoles are not a salient feature of polymyositis but are more suggestive of inclusion body myositis.

36. D (Chapter 10.III.B)   Perifascicular atrophy is the most salient pathologic feature of dermatomyositis.

37. C (Chapter 1.I.B)   Rosenthal fibers are frequently seen in all the listed conditions except fibrillary astrocytoma.

38. D (Chapter 2.II.A)   Cerebral blood flow constitutes about 20% of cardiac output.

39. D (Chapter 3.I.B)   Trisomy 22 is generally not a feature of diffuse astrocytomas.

40. B (Chapter 4.I.D)   Compression of the posterior cerebral artery in lateral transtentorial herniation may result in an infarct of the calcarine cortex.

41. B (Chapter 5.I.B)   The constellation of findings listed is classic for Dandy-Walker syndrome.

42. D (Chapter 9.II.F)   A Ziehl-Neelsen stain is the most useful one listed in identifying mycobacterial organisms.

43. E (Chapter 6.II.A)   Metachromatic leukodystrophy is the result of an arylsulfatase A deficiency (autosomal recessive on chromosome 22q). Arcuate fibers are preserved and white matter macrophages are filled with sulfatides.

44. B (Chapter 8.III.J)   The CERAD criteria are based on a semiquantitative assessment of plaque frequency in the neocortex.

45. A (Chapter 10.III.B)   Most patients with dermatomyositis respond well to steroid or immunosuppressive therapy.

46. A (Chapter 5.I.C)   A LIS-1 gene defect is associated with the development of Miller-Dieker syndrome agyria.

47. E (Chapter 9.II.I)   Demyelination is not a typical feature of meningovascular syphilitic disease.

48. B (Chapter 10.III.C)   The etiology of inclusion body myositis remains unknown.

49. A (Chapter 1.I.B)   Alzheimer type II astrocytes may be prominently seen in hepatic diseases marked by elevated ammonia levels.

50. B (Chapter 2.II.D)   Macrophage infiltration in an infarct begins at about 24 hr.

51. C (Chapter 3.I.F)   Glioblastoma multiforme is the most common glioma type.

52. B (Chapter 4.II.A)   Epidural hemorrhage is associated with rupture of the middle meningeal artery.

53. D (Chapter 5.I.C)   Cortical dysplasia is not associated with neurofibromatosis type II.

54. A (Chapter 6.II.B)   Globoid cell leukodystrophy is the result of a deficiency of galactocerebroside-B galactosidase.

55. C (Chapter 8.IV.M)   Bunina bodies are more typically seen in amyotrophic lateral sclerosis. Lewy bodies may be encountered in a subset of Alzheimer's patients.

56. A (Chapter 9.III.B)   Cryptococcus is a budding yeast with a thick mucopolysaccharide wall.

57. C (Chapter 9.III.E)   The features described are most likely attributable to Mucormycosis.

58. C (Chapter 5.I.D)   Lissencephaly or agyria is associated with developmental abnormalities which occur during the 11th–13th wk of gestation.

59. C (Chapter 9.III.G)   A protoplasmic body is seen in Blastomycosis infection (fungal infection).

60. E (Chapter 8.III.K)   Infarcts of >100 mL volume are associated with the clinical development of dementia.

61. C (Chapter 1.I.C)   The "fried egg" appearance of oligodendrocytes is related to delays in formalin fixation (an artifact).

62. D (Chapter 2.II.E)   The least common site for a lacunar infarct is in the mamillary bodies.

63. E (Chapter 3.I.F) Perinecrotic pseudopalisading is a feature more commonly observed in glioblastoma multiforme than metastatic carcinoma.

64. C (Chapter 4.II.B) About 50% of acute subdural hematomas are associated with a skull fracture.

65. E (Chapter 5.I.D) The features described are most characteristic of the Walker-Warburg syndrome.

66. E (Chapter 6.II.C) Most forms of adrenoleukodystrophy are X-linked.

67. D (Chapter 10.IV.A) Target fibers are associated with neurogenic atrophy.

68. A (Chapter 11.II.C) Diphtheritic neuropathy is a demyelinative neuropathy related primarily to Schwann cell dysfunction.

69. D (Chapter 8.III.E) Silver stains (bodian) are useful in highlighting neurofibrillary tangles.

70. B (Chapter 8.IV.B) The huntington gene is located on chromosome 4p.

71. C (Chapter 9.III.I) Actinomycosis bacteria are associated with sulfur granule formation.

72. A (Chapter 9.IV.A) Poliovirus more typically results in Cowdry type B inclusions.

73. D (Chapter 1.I.D) Blepharoplasts are the ciliary body attachments in ependymal cells.

74. C (Chapter 2.III.A) Approximately 20% of saccular aneurysms are bilateral.

75. B (Chapter 3.I.J) Eosinophilic granular bodies are observed in a majority of pilocytic astrocytomas.

76. B (Chapter 4.II.C) Traumatic basilar subarachnoid hemorrhages are related to vertebral artery tears.

77. D (Chapter 5.I.E) A brain weight of 2350 g would represent megaloencephaly.

78. E (Chapter 6.II.C) All of the organs listed may contain inclusions in adrenoleukodystrophy except for the pancreas.

79. A (Chapter 9.IV.A) Granulomatous inflammation is not a typical feature of viral infections in the CNS.

80. B (Chapter 9.IV.G) Most patients with SSPE die from the disease.

81. B (Chapter 10.IV.B) Fascicular atrophy is commonly encountered in muscle biopsies of patients with spinal muscular atrophy, including Kugelberg-Welander disease.

82. E (Chapter 8.IV.B) Huntington's chorea is a trinucleotide (CAG) repeat disorder.

83. D (Chapter 11.III.A) Morton's neuroma arises associated with the interdigital nerve of the foot at intermetatarsal sites.

84. C (Chapter 9.IV.I) Negri bodies are intraneuronal cytoplasmic inclusions.

85. C (Chapter 1.I.E) Microglial cells are HAM56 positive.

86. A (Chapter 2.III.A) Tuberous sclerosis is not associated with the development of saccular aneurysms.

87. E (Chapter 3.I.M) Increased mitotic activity is not a feature of the typical pleomorphic xanthoastrocytoma.

88. A (Chapter 3.VIII.B) The Langerhan's cell histiocytes stain with CD1a.

89. B (Chapter 4.III.D) Raccoon eyes (periorbital ecchymoses) are associated with basilar skull fractures.

90. B (Chapter 5.I.G) Narrowing of the superior temporal gyrus is seen in Down's syndrome.

91. A (Chapter 6.II.D) Megalencephaly is a common feature of Alexander's disease.

92. B (Chapter 8.IV.B) Vonsattel grade I lesions of Huntington's chorea are grossly normal with up to 50% neuronal loss in the striatum and gliosis in the caudate and putamen.

93. D (Chapter 9.IV.J) Retrograde axoplasmic transport is associated with herpes virus.

94. C (Chapter 5.I.J) Sommer sector (CA1), CA4, and the dentate are the areas most severely affected (neuronal loss and gliosis) in hippocampal sclerosis.

95. C (Chapter 10.IV.C) Myasthenia gravis is characterized by the presence of circulating antibodies to the acetylcholine receptor.

96. A (Chapter 11.III.B) Guillian-Barre syndrome is not associated with HLA B27.

97. D (Chapter 1.I.H) Layer III of the cerebral cortex is known as the outer pyramidal layer.

98. A (Chapter 2.III.C) Dolichoectasia (elongation, widening, and tortuosity of the artery) is associated with the formation of fusiform aneurysms.

99. D (Chapter 3.I.U) Necrosis is distinctly uncommon in gangliogliomas.

100. D (Chapter 3.X.A) Paraganglioma is composed of cells arranged in nests or lobules referred to as zellballen.

101. C (Chapter 4.V.A) The wounding capacity of a gunshot wound is most related to the velocity of the bullet.

102. C (Chapter 5.II.G) Periventricular coagulative necrosis in a premature infant is termed periventricular leukomalacia.

103. D (Chapter 9.IV.L) Congenital CMV infection does not result in megalencephaly.

104. B (Chapter 10.IV.D) Enhanced neurotransmission with repeated stimulation is seen with Lambert-Eaton syndrome.

105. A (Chapter 3.X.D) Cholesterol accounts for the "motor oil" quality of craniopharyngioma cyst fluid.

106. E (Chapter 11.III.D) Leprosy neuropathy is not a toxin-mediated process.

107. D (Chapter 8.IV.C) Autosomal dominant transmission of Parkinson's disease is linked with the α-synuclein gene.

108. A (Chapter 10.V.B) Nemaline rods are derived from α-actinin or Z-band material.

109. C (Chapter 1.I.H) The pencil bundles of Wilson are thin fascicles of myelinated fibers seen in the caudate and putamen.

110. B (Chapter 2.III.B) Aspergillus is the most common cause of mycotic (fungal) aneurysms.

111. A (Chapter 3.II.B) Chromosome 1p and 19q deletions have been associated with chemoresponsiveness in oligodendrogliomas.

112. D (Chapter 4.V.B) Blunt head injury sustained in a landslide is an example of static loading.

113. D (Chapter 5.II.O) The least likely site of bilirubin deposition in kernicterus is in the claustrum.

114. C (Chapter 6.II.E) Canavan's disease is caused by a deficiency in aspartoacylase.

115. B (Chapter 10.V.A) Most congenital myopathies are nonprogressive or only slowly progressive.

116. B (Chapter 11.III.D) Lyme disease is acquired from a tick bite.

117. C (Chapter 8.IV.C) The ubiquitin immunostain can be useful in identifying Lewy bodies.

118. E (Chapter 9.IV.M) Oligodendroglial cell Cowdry A inclusions are characteristic of PML.

119. B (Chapter 9.IV.N) The term "vacuolar myelopathy" is used to described HIV-associated spinal cord changes.

120. E (Chapter 10.VI.A) Ragged red fibers are associated with mitochondrial abnormalities and are generally not seen with central core disease.

121. E (Chapter 1.I.H) The endplate of the hippocampus is designated CA4.

122. C (Chapter 2.IV.D) Cavernous angiomas are characterized by back-to-back vessels.

123. B (Chapter 3.II.E) The prognosis of central neurocytoma is good. Most patients live well beyond 2 yr of diagnosis.

124. D (Chapter 4.IV.B) A burst lobe represents a form of contrecoup contusion.

125. E (Chapter 5.III.A) The neurofibromin gene (neurofibromatosis type I) is located on chromosome 17q.

126. A (Chapter 6.II.F) A relative perivascular white matter sparing (tigroid demyelination) in characteristic of Pelizaeus-Merzbacher disease.

127. D (Chapter 9.IV.O) Viral inclusions are not seen with HTLV-1 infection.

128. B (Chapter 11.III.E) Paraneoplastic neuropathy is most often encountered with lung carcinoma (especially small cell carcinoma).

129. B (Chapter 8.IV.C) Lewy bodies are intraneuronal cytoplasmic inclusions.

130. B (Chapter 10.VI.A) Acromegaly is not associated with Kearns-Sayre syndrome.

131. B (Chapter 8.IV.E) The features described are characteristic of progressive supranuclear palsy.

132. C (Chapter 10.VI.B) Type II glycogenosis (acid maltase deficiency) is caused by a chromosome 17q defect.

133. A (Chapter 1.II.D) Ischemia-related perifascicular atrophy is a feature of dermatomyositis.

134. D (Chapter 2.V.A) Hypertension is the most common cause of nontraumatic hemorrhage.

135. E (Chapter 3.III.B) Extent of surgical resection is the most important factor in predicting outcome in ependymomas.

136. A (Chapter 4.V.C) Midbrain is the least common site (listed) of diffuse axonal injury.

137. B (Chapter 5.III.A) One plexiform neurofibroma is a major criterion for the diagnosis of neurofibromatosis type I.

138. D (Chapter 3.III.E) Mucoid stroma (mucin positive) is a distinguishing feature of myxopapillary ependymoma. All of the other features may be observed in ordinary ependymomas.

139. A (Chapter 9.V.A) Abscess is the most common pathologic manifestation of Toxoplasmosis infection in adults who are immunocompromised.

140. B (Chapter 10.VI.B)   Glycogen storage diseases are typically vacuolar myopathies.

141. D (Chapter 9.V.C)   Dhrcks nodes (foci of necrosis rimmed by microglia) are a feature of malaria.

142. B (Chapter 8.IV.F)   Hallervorden-Spatz disease is an autosomal recessive condition.

143. A (Chapter 9.V.D)   Cysticercosis is caused by the pork tapeworm (*Taenia solium*).

144. C (Chapter 11.III.E)   Anti-MAG antibodies are encountered in 50–90% of cases of dysproteinemic neuropathy.

145. D (Chapter 1.II.G)   The sarcomere runs from Z band to Z band.

146. E (Chapter 2.V.A)   Amyloid angiopathy is not associated with Pick's disease; it is associated with Alzheimer's disease.

147. A (Chapter 3.IV.A)   Metaplastic meningiomas are less likely to recur than the other types listed.

148. D (Chapter 5.III.B)   The merlin gene of neurofibromatosis type II is located on chromosome 22.

149. C (Chapter 7.I.B)   Tay-Sachs disease is a result of a hexosaminidase A deficiency.

150. A (Chapter 10.VI.B)   Type V glycogenosis (McArdle's disease) is caused by myophosphorylase deficiency.

151. C (Chapter 10.VI.C)   An oil-red-O stain for lipid would be most useful in diagnosing carnitine deficiency (a lipid-storage myopathy).

152. D (Chapter 9.V.F)   *Trypanosoma cruzi* (*T. cruzi*) is the causative agent of Chagas disease.

153. E (Chapter 7.I.B)   Visceral organ involvement including hepatosplenomegaly is not a prominent feature of Tay-Sachs disease.

154. A (Chapter 8.IV.I)   Multisystem atrophy includes olivopontocerebellar atrophy, Shy-Drager syndrome, and striatonigral degeneration.

155. B (Chapter 9.VI.B)   Microglial nodules are not a feature of Creutzfeldt-Jakob disease.

156. B (Chapter 11.III.F)   Abnormalities on chromosomes 1, 17, and X are associated with Charcot-Marie-Tooth disease.

157. B (Chapter 1.II.B)   Increased central nuclei (normally <3–5% of all fibers) is not typically seen in neurogenic atrophy.

158. B (Chapter 2.VI.A)   Wegener's vasculitis is commonly associated with granulomatous inflammation.

159. E (Chapter 3.IV.A)   Deletions on chromosome 22 are the most common cytogenetic abnormality in meningioma.

160. C (Chapter 4.V.C)   Diffuse axonal injury is manifested by punctate or streak-like hemorrhages and retraction balls or spheroids.

161. C (Chapter 5.III.C)   The subependymal giant-cell astrocytoma is associated with tuberous sclerosis.

162. B (Chapter 7.I.D)   An accumulation of sphingomyelin and cholesterol as a result of sphingomyelinase deficiency is a feature of Niemann-Pick disease.

163. B (Chapter 8.IV.K)   The most common cause of death in Friedrich's ataxia is related to heart disease.

164. D (Chapter 8.IV.K)   Posterior column degeneration is commonly seen in Friedrich's ataxia.

165. C (Chapter 9.VI.A)   The prion protein gene is located on chromosome 20.

166. D (Chapter 10.VI.F)   Dilated sarcoplasmic reticulum and tubular aggregates are features of the periodic paralyses (channelopathies).

167. D (Chapter 11.III.F)   Nerve enlargement is a common finding in Dejerine-Sottas disease (HMSN III).

168. B (Chapter 11.III.G)   Refsum's disease is due to phytanoyl CoA α-hydroxylase deficiency.

169. B (Chapter 1.II.G)   Desmin filaments link Z discs together and join them to the plasmalemma.

170. A (Chapter 2.VI.A)   The leptomeningeal vessels are the highest yield area to look for vasculitis on a biopsy.

171. B (Chapter 3.IV.B)   Solitary fibrous tumors, in contrast to meningiomas, are generally CD34 positive.

172. E (Chapter 4.I.D)   Duret hemorrhages are midline brain stem hemorrhages associated with lateral transtentorial herniation.

173. A (Chapter 5.III.C)   Schwannoma is not associated with tuberous sclerosis.

174. C (Chapter 7.I.E)   Cherry red spots are not a salient feature of Gaucher's disease.

175. B (Chapter 10.VII.E)   Steroid myopathy is marked by a type IIb muscle fiber atrophy.

176. C (Chapter 3.VIII.A)   Most primary CNS lymphomas are diffuse large B-cell type (REAL classification).

177. C (Chapter 5.III.E)   von Hippel-Lindau is associated with hemangioblastoma, not hemangiopericytoma.

178. D (Chapter 11.III.H)   Vitamin E deficiency may manifest as spinocerebellar degeneration with a sensory neuropathy caused by fat malabsorption.

179. D (Chapter 8.IV.M)   SOD1 gene defect on chromosome 21 is associated with amyotrophic lateral sclerosis.

180. A (Chapter 8.IV.M)   Hirano bodies are not a frequent finding in amyotrophic lateral sclerosis.

181. C (Chapter 1.III.B)   Mast cells are normally present in the endoneurium in small numbers.

182. C (Chapter 2.VII.B)   The notch 3 gene of CADASIL is located on chromosome 19.

183. E (Chapter 3.IV.B)   Physaliphorous cells are a feature of chordoma.

184. E (Chapter 5.III.C)   Sturge-Weber disease is not an autosomal dominant condition.

185. C (Chapter 5.III.C)   A nevus flammeus (port wine stain) in the trigeminal region is associated with Sturge-Weber disease.

186. B (Chapter 7.I.D)   Sea blue histiocytes are a feature of Niemann-Pick disease.

187. E (Chapter 2.III.A)   Giant aneurysms are >2.5 cm in size.

188. A (Chapter 3.V.A)   The lateral ventricle is the most common site of origin of choroid plexus papilloma in children; 4th ventricle in adults.

189. B (Chapter 5.III.H)   The dysplastic cerebellar gangliocytoma (Lhermette-Duclos) is associated with Cowden syndrome.

190. B (Chapter 7.I.E)   Gaucher's disease is caused by glucocerebrosidase deficiency related to a defect on chromosome 1q.

191. C (Chapter 7.I.O)   Most patients with Leigh's disease die in the 1st decade of life.

192. E (Chapter 7.II.C)   Ethanol is not associated with neurofibrillary tangle formation.

193. D (Chapter 1.III.F)   The pi granules of Reich are lamellated structures that increase in number with increasing age in the Schwann cell cytoplasm.

194. A (Chapter 2.VII.D)   There is no amyloid deposition associated with moya moya.

195. B (Chapter 3.IV.E)   Hemangioblastoma may produce erythropoietin resulting in a secondary polycythemia vera.

196. B (Chapter 7.I.F)   The features described are characteristic of Batten's disease or the ceroid-lipofuscinoses.

197. E (Chapter 7.I.L)   All the features listed are salient features of Fabry's disease.

198. E (Chapter 7.I.N)   Lafora-body disease is associated with a chromosome 6q defect.

199. B (Chapter 8.IV.N)   The presentation is consistent with Werdnig-Hoffman disease associated with a chromosome 5 abnormality.

200. B (Chapter 1.III.J)   The best approximation of a myelinated : unmyelinated axon ratio is 1 : 4.

201. B (Chapter 9.IV.D)   Viral infections account for the majority of aseptic meningitis cases.

202. A (Chapter 9.VI.E)   Most patients with familial insomnia syndrome die within a few years of symptom onset.

203. A (Chapter 1.III.H)   Discontinuous saltatory conduction is most related to the nodes of Ranvier.

204. B (Chapter 2.III.A)   Absence of the media defines the saccular aneurysm.

205. C (Chapter 3.VI.C)   Medulloblastomas are associated with chromosome 17 alterations.

206. D (Chapter 3.VI.C)   Synaptophysin is the single best marker for medulloblastoma.

207. A (Chapter 3.VI.C)   Age <3 yr is associated with a poor prognosis in medulloblastoma.

208. A (Chapter 2.VI.A)   Erythrocyte sedimentation rates are often normal or only slight elevated in primary angiitis of the CNS.

209. E (Chapter 3.VII.A)   Melanotic schwannoma (often with psammoma bodies) is associated with Carney's complex.

210. D (Chapter 11.III.I)   Transthyretin (prealbumin) is related to hereditary amyloid neuropathy.

Bibliography

Birch, R., Bonney, G., Wynn Parry, C. B. (1998). Surgical Disorders of the Peripheral Nerves. Churchill Livingstone. Edinburgh.

Burger, P. C., Scheithauer, B. W. (1994). Tumors of the Central Nervous System. Armed Forces Institute of Pathology, Washington, DC.

Burger, P. C., Scheithauer, B. W., Vogel, F. S. (1991). Surgical Pathology of the Nervous System and Its Coverings. Churchill Livingstone, New York.

deGirolami, U., Anthony, D. C., Frosch, M. D. (1999). Peripheral nerve and skeletal muscle and the central nervous system. In: Pathologic Basis of Disease (Cotran, R. S., Kumar, V., Collins, T., eds), W.B. Saunders Co., Philadelphia.

Davis, R. L., Robertson, D. M. (eds.) (1999). Textbook of Neuropathology. Williams & Wilkins, Baltimore, MD.

Engel, A. G., Franzini-Armstrong, C. (eds.) (1993). Principles and Practice of Neuropathology. Mosby, St. Louis, MO.

Fuller, G. N., Burger, P. C. (1997). Central nervous system. In: Histology for Pathologists (Sternberg, S. S., ed.), Lippincott-Raven, Philadelphia.

Graham, D. I., Lantos, P. L. (eds.) (1997). Greenfield's Neuropathology. Oxford University Press, New York.

Kleihues, P., Cavenee, W. K. (eds.) (2000). Pathology and Genetics: Tumours of the Nervous System. IARC Press, Lyon, France

Loughlin, M. (1993). Muscle Biopsy. A Laboratory Investigation. Butterworth-Heinemann, Oxford.

Nelson, J. S., Parisi, J. E., Schochet, S. S., Jr. (eds.) (1993). Principles and Practice of Neuropathology. Mosby, St. Louis, MO.

Ortiz-Hidalgo, C., Weller, R. O. (1997). Peripheral nervous system. In: Histology for Pathologists (Sternberg, S. S., ed.). Lippincott-Raven, Philadelphia.

Prayson, R. A., Cohen, M. L. (2000). Practical Differential Diagnosis in Surgical Neuropathology. Humana Press, Totowa, NJ.

Schochet, S. S. Jr. (1986). Diagnostic Pathology of Skeletal Muscle and Nerve. Appleton-Century-Crofts, Norwalk, CT.

Vinters, H. V., Farrell, M. A., Mischel, P. S., Anders, K. H. (1998). Diagnostic Neuropathology. Marcel Dekker, Inc., New York.

INDEX